Health Tonics, Elixirs and Potions

for the

Look and Feel of Youth

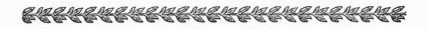

HEALTH TONICS, ELIXIRS and POTIONS
for the
LOOK and FEEL
of YOUTH

CARLSON WADE

Foreword by Amil J. Johnson, M.D.

PARKER PUBLISHING COMPANY, INC.   West Nyack, N.Y.

DEDICATION

To your renewed youth and
the best health-packed years of
your life.

Second Printing . . . . . April 1973

PRINTED IN THE UNITED STATES OF AMERICA
ISBN-0-13-384545-1
B & P

Foreword
by A Doctor of Medicine

In the search for a way to help awaken the hidden look and feel of youth for yourself, it is beneficial to seek the "fountains of youth" offered by Nature. "Live" food juices, health tonics, elixirs that are made from fresh fruits and vegetables, potions that are comprised of herbs, seeds, plants, are known to rejuvenate the body's physical and chemical processes and help put youthful glamour into your appearance and help check the aging factor to promote a "forever young" feeling.

In this commendable book, there is a veritable treasure of all-natural health tonics, potions and elixirs that make it tastefully enjoyable to help you regain the look and feel of youth.

It contains a great many simple yet effective recipes for tonics and health potions that benefit you by promoting improved and youthful digestion, a rejuvenated bloodstream and its circulation, more youthful gland action, revitalized body organs, and much more.

It is gratifying to see that the programs in the book utilize all-natural ingredients, easy to prepare right in your own home, and at no extra cost to you.

I highly recommend this book by Carlson Wade to those who seek better health, and a lifetime that is filled with the look and feel of youth.

AMIL J. JOHNSON, M.D.

3

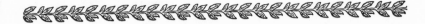

What This Book Can

Do for You

Throughout my many years as a medical reporter and writer of health articles and books, I have noted case histories reporting "health miracles" brought about through the drinking of all-natural health tonics, various selected fruit and vegetable juices, plant-herbal elixirs and potions. These reports told of how distressing common ailments that prematurely age a person, such as arthritic pains, sagging skin, faulty digestion, chronic fatigue, sleeplessness, and sluggish kidney-liver functioning, were overcome through a program of drinking selected all-natural liquids and special combinations of such health tonics. Such a program was also able to help promote the look and feeling of youthfulness.

This book has gathered together many such programs, and shows you how to use Nature's special "Fountain of Youth" liquids for internal use and help stimulate the look and feel of youth for you at any age. You need no longer feel that you may have "lost" your youthfulness in our vibrantly youthful world. The "secret" of renewing youthfulness is increasing the power of your body's metabolism. Certain fresh fruit, vegetable and other natural juices and liquids, taken in proper combination, can work wonders in activating this key power for your looking and feeling more youthful.

By using the tonics, elixirs and potions as programmed in this book, you will be able to help build for yourself a "young feeling," a "look of youthfulness," and a more youthful attitude and personality that will be noticed and appreciated by others.

When you drink the all-natural health preparations as worked out for you in this book, they go to work for you promptly. They speedily start correcting the internal causes that may be dragging you down to premature aging. They help melt the harsh aging signs that make you look and feel unnecessarily older.

Each chapter in this book contains experiences of those who have followed the programs for youthfulness and how they have been able thereby to have a more youthfully satisfying life.

The programs and guidance in this book are completely medicine-less. They involve no drugs, nor expensive things for you to buy. All ingredients can be purchased quite economically in your local supermarket or health food store.

No doubt, many of these ingredients for health tonics, elixirs and potions are already in your refrigerator and pantry. It will be a simple matter, and a healthfully happy experience, for you to follow the easy programs in this book for a healthfully regenerated life having the look and feel of youth.

CARLSON WADE

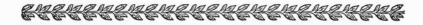

Contents

How a Natural Juice Recharges the Arteries with
Youth • How Seed Oils Promote a Cholesterol-
Washing Benefit • The Liquid Food that Extended
Youthful Life • Why Healthy Arteries Are the Pipe-
lines of Youth • How Lecithin Promoted Arterial
Rejuvenation in Two "Over-40" Patients • How An
"Energy Elixir" Promotes Internal Rejuvenation

How Liquid Fasting Rejuvenates Five Health Systems
• How Jane E. Plans Her One-Day "All Liquid"
Youth-Restoration Program • How to Begin a Controlled
Fasting Program • How to End a Controlled Fasting
Program

How to Make Herbal Teas • Herbal Teas for Mind-
Body Power: A Listing—with Their Benefits

Nature's Foods: A List—with Their Benefits • Three
Benefits of Live Food Juices for Added Youthful

Health Tonics, Elixirs and Potions

for the

Look and Feel of Youth

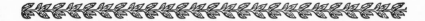

Chapter 1

Proof that Natural Liquid Foods

Can Awaken Your Hidden Youthfulness

NATURE wants you to enjoy a lifetime of Young Feeling. Nature wants you to be spared the age-inducing illnesses and unnecessary mind-body decline. Nature wants you to live healthfully and to look youthfully, as well. In order to benefit from Nature's plan to give you a Young Feeling, she has prepared a Garden of Health in which grow the sources of effervescent youthfulness and natural healing. In this Garden of Health grow the 'secrets" of how you can look and feel young at any age. The "secrets" are the *live food juices* that lie within healthful raw fruits, vegetables, grains, herbs, roots, plants of every description.

These *live food juices* are liquid foods prepared by Nature, endowed with the power of almost all known (and many yet-unknown) nutrients that create internal-external nourishment to help revive-rejuvenate-replenish the mind-body organism to promote the sought-after Look and Feel of Youth.

The "secret" is in the *live food juices* of Nature's own foods in the Garden of Health. This book is your guide to discovering the different *live food juices* that are Nature's keys to unlock your hidden wellsprings of bubbling health and thereby awaken your hidden look and feel of youth.

HOW RUTH W. USED LIQUID FOODS TO TURN BACK THE "AGING CLOCK"

Schoolteacher Ruth W. woke up mornings as tired as when she dragged herself to bed the night before. Looking at her reflection in the mirror, she saw a line-filled face, dull eyes, and pale complexion. Moving around as she dressed, Ruth W. felt stiffening of her muscles, a knife-sharp pain in her lower back when she bent over to tie her shoelaces, and a sense of vertigo (dizzyness) when she straightened up again. Ruth W. was an "old" woman at just 41.

Processed Foods Were Responsible for Premature Aging. Ruth W. was an habitual processed food consumer. Everything was prepared, pre-cooked, even pre-table set in the convenient "cook in the package" plastic tray she picked up at a supermarket. These so-called foods were "dead" foods that had been depleted of vital nutrients that help perpetuate a look-feel young biology. Ruth W. was actually eating herself into premature and unnecessary old age.

Chance Remark Overheard Calls for Action. It was during a parent-teacher meeting, when Ruth W. brought her young child to the auditorium, that something happened. A well-meaning newcomer observed that Ruth W. was a fortunate "grandmother" to have such a lovely "grandchild." It was the first time anyone had voiced an opinion about her age. Here she was a young mother, but she was mistaken for a grand-mother! She bit back the tears and moved on to several exhibits that had been arranged by local merchants for this special parent-teacher meeting. She found herself standing before an exhibit that offered freshly prepared live food juices. The benefit of these juices, it was explained, is in the non-processed treasure of youth-building nutrients. Since vitamins, minerals, enzymes, and other valuable body building blocks are destroyed during processing, it is essential to obtain them in Nature-created foods. A glass of freshly squeezed juices was offered to Ruth W. for a sample taste of Young Feeling food.

Live Food Juices Help Restore Look and Feel of Youth. Just one glass of a fruit cocktail beverage made Ruth W. feel better. She decided to try it when the exhibitor said that many other "grandmothers" reported feeling so much younger with freshly squeezed juices. She purchased the electric juice extractor and thus began her program:

1. *Morning.* Emphasis is upon fresh fruit juices with their rich source of Vitamin C and skin-tissue building *collagen* which helps bind together, repair and rejuvenate the millions of body cells that promote a look and feel of youth. At least two glasses of freshly squeezed fruit juices before breakfast.

2. *Noontime.* Emphasis is upon fresh vegetable juices with a powerful source of minerals needed to enrich the bloodstream, regulate hormonal health, stimulate glandular function, help to stimulate youth-building life processes. At least two glasses of freshly squeezed vegetable juices before lunch.

3. *Dinnertime.* Beverages consisting of herbal teas, seed oils for raw vegetable salads, plus the juice of *one* selected vegetable. The benefit here is to have an enriched supply of youth-building nutrients from just *one* plant of Nature, so it can help create rejuvenation with little interference.

THE CORRECTIVE FOOD PROGRAM THAT PUT RUTH W. ON THE PATHWAY TO THE GARDEN OF YOUTH

Ruth W. enjoyed a partial revitalization. She felt more energetic in the morning and she felt a slightly less poignant pain when bending over. But she still looked crease-lined, although the deep shadows were less severe. Now she realized that she had followed only one portion of Nature's plan. She had improved her health with the nutrients found in live food juices, but she continued to deny herself all of Nature's benefits because she still used processed foods with nearly all meals. She went about with these changes:

1. *All fruits and vegetables were to be fresh.* The benefit here is that fruits and vegetables are brimming with precious and perishable nutrients that help promote the look and feel of youth. *Vitamins* nourish the skin and vital body organs. *Minerals* regulate water balance, strengthen skeletal system, revitalize a sluggish hormone system. *Proteins* build and repair tissues and cells and are of prime importance in nourishing a Young Again feeling. *Enzymes* are the body's miracle workers, creating a youthful metabolism, scouring the body of accumulated wastes, creating the valuable metabolic systems of body rejuvenation. *Unsaturated fatty acids* are needed to promote a resilient arterial network of young transportation media within the body. These precious nutrients are largely destroyed during processing. So Ruth W. substituted *fresh* fruits and vegetables that were rich in these youth-restorating nutrients.

2. *Natural sweets helped improve assimilation of nutrients.* Ruth W. eliminated all artificial sweeteners; she eliminated white sugar in any form and that included foods that were made with white sugar. This non-food has an internal corrosive-acid action and dissolves and even destroys the perishable nutrients that are introduced through liquid foods. In their place, Ruth W. selected mineral-rich honey, Vitamin C-rich rose hips powder (sold at most health food stores), fresh date powder and appropriate herbs and spices. She had learned that you cannot compromise with Nature. To reap the rewards of the look-feel youth quality of liquid foods, she had to flatter them by giving up harsh non-foods such as sugars.

3. *Digestive power was revitalized by utilization of natural seed oils.* Ruth W. gave up her so-called hard fats because when used in cooking, they often created internal chain molecules that rendered difficult digestion. She used natural seed oils. These could be made from peanuts, safflower seed,

corn, wheat germ, or any other all-natural source. (Coconut oil is inadvisable because of its extremely high fatty acid content.) She learned that foods and liquids consumed are essential to health but that *assimilation* is the core of the Young Again program. With seed oils flattering digestion, the nutrients in juices and natural foods could work without interference.

4. *A freshly squeezed live food juice just one hour before each of the three daily meals, helps nourish the digestive-assimilation program for better youth.* The body processes become refreshed-rejuvenated with the stream of youth-building nutrients in fresh live food juices. Drink one glass just one hour before your meals to help promote a better internal tonus of the digestive system. This facilitates assimilation.

5. *Eat non-processed foods for living health.* Mrs. Ruth W. eliminated all packaged, processed, pre-cooked "foods" which were actually "dead" foods. Small wonder she was actually eating herself to premature aging! In their place, she selected fresh meats, fish, poultry, eggs, cheeses, rich in the life-youth giving qualities of Nature. With this program, she was soon on the way to recovery, so to speak. She had actually turned back the "aging clock" through all-natural foods with emphasis on liquid foods.

Ruth W. Becomes a Young Mother Again. Two months of the natural program with emphasis upon liquid foods made Ruth W. feel and enjoy restored youth. Now, when she attended a scout meeting with her daughter, she was mistaken for her "older sister." It was a flattering mistake—thanks be to Nature's live food juices.

SEVEN WAYS IN WHICH LIQUID FOODS CREATE MIRACLE YOUTH

Nutritional gerontologists (scientists who relate nutrition to aging disorders) have found that the process of aging is *not* so mysterious after all. They have learned that so-called aging is often traced to seven basic causes. By applying corrective nutrition with emphasis upon raw live juices, they reportedly succeeded in helping to promote invigoration and a feeling of youthful health in many persons.

Here are the reported seven ways in which liquid foods in the form of *live food juices* are able to help stimulate the body processes that maintain and restore a look and feel of youth:

1. *Raw juices have a built-in "self-timing" device that improves nutritional youth.* The so-called sluggish and declining state of health is often attributed to improper eating practices. Overeating, for instance, increases the heart action and causes a fast pumping; this increases the blood supply for added body weight and resultant high blood pressure. This may cause degeneration of tissues of the heart and brain. With earliest symptoms of sluggishness, there is a general run-down feeling and a sign of declining youth. Raw fruit and vegetable juices do not overwork or overtax the system because they cannot be over-consumed. You drink until satisfied and then drink no more. This eases heart action, spares extra digestive labor and thus creates a feeling of relaxed and vitalic youth. You cannot really "overeat" with fresh raw juices that help control the rapacious appetite.

2. *Improve the youthful health of your genetic inheritance with fresh live food juices.* The key to prolonged and restored youth lies in the body's genetic makeup. Genes are situated in or on the chromosomes; these are thread or rod-like substances that are visible under a microscope. They actually determine your youthful appearance and health. The tiny microscopic filaments of genes are nourished by enzymes as well as vitamins and minerals such as those found in fresh live juices. By nourishing your genes with live food juices, you help rebuild the core of your very life and health.

3. *Radiation and pollution may be eased by rebuilding resistance through corrective nutrition.* Most people accumulate small amounts of age-causing radiation during a lifetime. There are atmospheric X-rays caused by nuclear testing as well as X-rays given by a physician. Often, this radiation attacks the body cells and tissues. Because they absorb these

rays, cells may alter and age signs may appear in very early life. Live food juices are rich in enzymes and vitamins needed to rebuild and strengthen the billions of body cells and tissues. This helps resist the ravages of radiation-caused unnecessary aging problems.

4. *Fresh juices help nourish, sustain and prolong the life of vital cells in the body.* Daily, millions of cells disintegrate and die. Nature then needs vitamins, minerals, enzymes and amino acids to help replace them. These vital cellular-nourishing nutrients are abundant in live food juices. A deficiency of such nutrients may lead to such serious tissue depletion that "old age" may be seen at just 30.

5. *Juice extractives help promote cellular sustenance.* Nutrients in live food juices help body cells maintain a healthful biochemical rhythm. Incorrect cellular reproduction is one contributing cause to body breakdown. Just as cells die every day, other body cells split and multiply. If a cell splits wrongly, it may become useless or, more seriously, it could become malignant and cause health depletion. Live food juices furnish the healing substances that help promote cellular sustenance and normal regularity.

6. *Liquid foods help "lubricate" the body's arterial network.* Unsaturated fatty acids found in fresh cold-pressed vegetable seed oils are recognized for their power in helping to lubricate a stiffening of connective tissue. When tissues become inflexible, they may interfere with blood flow. Joints do not work. Skin sags. Food materials cannot easily pass through the hardened tissues and the body is denied the strength it needs for youthful help. Liquid oils are able to permeate the clogged tissues and help to lubricate the connective network to promote youthful flexibility. Fresh juices also help transport much-needed nourishment to the body when solids cannot pass through the clogged organism.

7. *Juices offer "buffering" action to age-causing stress situations.* Many people lose the bloom of youth after a "stress" situation. Now, stress situations occur from outside forces such as bruised bones in earlier years, a serious illness, and recurring symptoms. There are stress situations that

occur from internal sources such as emotional tension and environmental attacks. All of these stress syndromes bring on premature aging. Noise and air pollution as well as excessive sunshine also lead to forms of aging. Fresh juices are especially needed because of the minerals that offer a "buffering" action to help soothe the onslaughts of stress from within and without. The rich sources of Nature's nutrients help encourage your internal wellsprings of youth to gush forth with resistance to the ravages of our civilization.

HOW JANET Y. DEFIED "HEREDITY" AND ENJOYED RENEWED YOUTH

Janet Y. at age 37 should have been healthy, bubbling over with joyful enthusiasm. The problem is that she came from a long line of ancestors who had allergies, chronic cold catching, severe migraine headaches and susceptibility to any age-causing illness that came upon the scene. Janet Y. was resigned to her fate when she saw her sisters and brothers were all victims of various nagging illnesses; they felt and looked old. So did she.

A Severe Sore Throat Alerts Janet to Youth-Powers of Raw Juices. When Janet Y. caught one of her recurring sore throats and was confined to bed, she went on a juice program because she was unable to swallow solid foods. She consumed huge quantities of freshly squeezed fruit and vegetable juices. She also followed a local "folk remedy" of two tablespoons of apple cider vinegar mixed with one glass of freshly squeezed orange juice and a teaspoon of honey for palatability. This mixture was a powerhouse of vitamins, minerals, and enzymes that helped combat the infectious wastes that led to her respiratory distress. Together with a program of fresh raw juices, she supercharged her body with nutrients and did more than recover from this mild flu bout. She actually looked and felt younger.

She decided to include juices in her daily food program; doing so, she was able to defy "heredity" and was able to build internal resistance to age-causing illnesses. She scoffed at the tale that "illness runs in the family" and soon lost the leathery skin and flaky thin dandruff; she developed a lovely peach glow and dark, resilient, shining hair. Enzymes in live juices promoted a natural and healthful hormonal flow and she became the "young" member of the family; in reality, she was older than the others who still scoffed, but envied her as they saw how Nature could help her become youthfully healthy.

WHY JUICES ARE MORE BENEFICIAL
THAN SOLID FOODS

It has been noted that fresh juices exert more benefits in helping to stimulate the hidden power of youth than solid fruits and vegetables. Of course, your corrective food program should include healthful fruits and vegetables as a base. But juices have been seen to provide the following benefits that may be absent in solids:

1. EASY DIGESTION. Many of the precious "building materials" and vitamins are found in the juices; these are locked within the cellulose fibers of the plant. In order to take out these nutrients, the digestive system must labor to break down the fibrous cells. For many digestive systems, this may be a difficult task. Raw juices contain "instant digestion" of such nutrients that might otherwise remain locked within the cellulose fibers and imprisoned until passed off.

2. SPEEDY ASSIMILATION. In the form of juice, it is said that the system can assimilate over 90% of the youth-building elements. Ordinarily, it may take up to four hours to assimilate bulk food. But a glass of natural juice, with fibrous bulk removed, is assimilated and in use by the body within 10 to 20 minutes. It is this power of juices that helps promote the much sought-after look and feel of youth. What you eat is vital but what you assimilate is inviolate! Juices provide the speedy assimilation that digestion may not always provide.

3. NATURE DOES YOUR CHEWING FOR YOU. Many who suffer from disturbances of the digestive tract or have chewing problems, find it difficult to eat roughage-containing foods. But by means of juicing your fruits and vegetables, Nature does the chewing! This means that you no longer need deny yourself the benefits of nutrients locked in tough fibrous plant foods because of chewing problems. A juice extractor helps break down these fibers, release the nutrients, and offer you a glass of youthful health—chewed by Nature!

4. JUICES CONTAIN HIDDEN-SECRET YOUTH FACTORS. If there is a miracle in the youth-building power of raw juices, it may be in the hidden-secret and as yet unknown factors found in plant foods. Many nutrients are known, but many are *not* known. These youth factors are believed to be present in plant foods and by extracting the juices, they are released and make available the easily-digested substances that you need.

5. DRINK FROM NATURE'S FOUNTAIN. Plants provide you with sun-enriched juice foods. When we consider that plant foods have been naturally created by solar energy, that they contain the life-giving elements that the sun and the mineral-rich earth have buried deep into their fiber cells, we may well recognize this discovery: that when we take the juices from the cells of these plant foods with *no* processing of any kind, we immediately put their beneficial fluids into our bodies. This enables us to drink from Nature's fountain, benefiting in a youthful physical and mental objective.

6. PROMOTES YOUTH FROM WITHIN. To look and feel young, begin with your internal structure! *You will look and feel as young as your insides.* Live plant juices are youth-builders with their powerhouse of natural nutrients that have not been changed by heating. These plant juices are absorbed directly into the bloodstream to nourish the entire body. Plant juices are able to be utilized even by the weakest digestive system. You can rebuild youth through a nourished digestive system made youthful through plant juices.

7. FEEL YOUNG WITH PLANT JUICES. The British Ministry of Health and Public Health Service Laboratory lauds plant

juices by saying: "The sources of the essential amino acids, the cell building factors, are destroyed by heat and processing and not obtainable in foods thus prepared; juices, therefore, are the only means practical to get these rebuilding factors.

Relieves Disorders. "Juices are valuable in relief of hypertension, cardiovascular and kidney diseases and obesity. Good results have also been obtained in rheumatic, degenerative and toxic states. Juices have all-around protective action. Good results can be obtained in large amounts up to one litre (quart) daily in treatment of peptic ulceration, also in treatment of chronic diarrhea, colitis and toxemia of gastric and intestinal origin.

Gently Soothing. "The high-buffering capacities of the juices reveal that they are very valuable in the treatment of hyper-chlorhydria. Milk has often been used for this purpose, but spinach juices, juices of cabbage, kale and parsley were far superior to milk for this purpose."[1] Plant juices acted as an internal "gyroscope" in that they helped stabilize a normal acid-alkaline digestive system.

SWISS DOCTOR HEALS PATIENTS WITH PLANT JUICES. The famed Dr. M. Bircher-Benner, who heads a sanatorium in the Swiss Alps, also uses plant juices for healing of his patients. Here is what Dr. Bircher-Benner has to say:[2]

"Juices are far superior to a milk diet. They are invaluable against diseases of metabolism such as gout and obesity. What is aimed at in such cases is the temporary reduction of food to a minimum in order to obtain the combustion of fat, to neutralize the poisoning effects of uric acid and to bring about its excretion. Anyone who understands how to observe such cases will be convinced of the astonishing nutritive power of this food.

"These nutritive juices are, as it were, the 'mother's milk' of those who are seriously ill, the only food they are still able to take. But they are not to be considered as mere beverages. The patient is *not* to drink them. He is to *eat* them. One small

---

[1]See: Dr. Max Bircher-Benner, *Food Science for All;* Bern, Switzerland.
[2]Dr. Bircher-Benner, *Food Science for All.*

spoonful after another is to be taken and slowly swallowed."

Dr. Bircher-Benner has healed thousands of people in his sanatorium in Switzerland by means of using live plant juices as part of the Look and Feel of Youth Program. Now, such a health-boosting program may be carried out right in your own home. You need not wait until the ravages of internal and external aging have taken their toll. You should take care of your health while you have it; nurture it and help it blossom into youthful feeling. Plant juices offer you that opportunity with the rich supply of working materials that might otherwise be unavailable.

HOW TO OBTAIN PLANT JUICES

You can obtain plant juices by means of any of the following:

1. *Juice Extractor is Best.* An electric juice extractor, such as those sold in almost all health food stores and housewares outlets, is regarded as the best source. An electric model is able to separate the juice from the pulp in a matter of minutes. The juice comes down a funnel right into your glass, for your healthful enjoyment. Visit any health store and make your selection of your preferred juice extractor.

2. *Manual Juicer.* There are many such manual juicers available in health stores as well as housewares outlets. You will have to press a lever to get the juice out of the plant and it may be too strenuous for some people. Nevertheless, it does the job of extracting juices from inserted fruits and vegetables and it may be satisfactory to many of you.

3. *Hand Squeeze Through Cheesecloth.* In the absence of a juicer (for example, when you are travelling), you may make your own juice in this simple manner. Cut up the fruit or vegetable into small pieces. Wrap in some clean cheesecloth. Twist and squeeze the juice out into a glass.

4. *Bottled Juices.* Because pasteurization and preservation require a pre-heating process, many valuable and perishable nutrients, such as enzymes, are depleted. It is this pre-cooking

process that makes bottled juices a lesser process that is destructive of nutrients. But you will obtain an appreciable and highly beneficial amount of valuable youthful nutrients by purchasing organic juices in health stores. Many such bottled and canned juices have not been subjected to pre-heating and are non-pasteurized so they do represent a storehouse of the valuable nutrients you need in your Look and Feel Young Program. Surely, a glass of these juices will help you when natural squeezed juices are unavailable.

Note: Because there are so many different electric juicers, it is impossible to list here the instructions for operation. Ask for a demonstration when contemplating purchase of a machine. Some suggestions would include the following.

Begin by purchasing fresh fruits and vegetables. Select organic-grown plant foods, wherever possible, such as those sold in a health store. Store in a refrigerator to help prevent loss of vitamin and mineral supply. When using raw foods, cut out all wilted or discolored spots. These should *not* be used since they may cause "juice fermentation" and loss of nutrient. Wash all plant foods beneath free flowing faucet water. Use a stiff vegetable brush to "scrub" away any residue.

Slice the plant into small pieces that can be inserted easily into the feeder of the juicer. Close the lid or whatever is used. Press the switch. Keep inserting the pieces in accordance with manufacturer's instructions. The juice will come down the spigot into the glass you should have waiting. Drink it on the spot.

Use Plant Pulp for Salads. The cellulose fibrous plant pulp may be used for salads; they need not be discarded. Scrape off with a spoon and put in a bowl. Season with a bit of seed oil (for vegetable pulp) or lemon juice (fruit pulp) and you have a nourishing salad. No waste.

How to Store Plant Juices. If you must store juices, use a glass bottle. Screw on a tight cap. Store in a section of your refrigerator where you keep milk. This helps to reduce any nutrient loss.

Keep Your Juicer in Sparkling Clean Condition. The woody

fibers of many plant foods may cling to the basin portion of the juicer. It is advisable to use warm water and a brush immediately after you have finished squeezing the juice. Keep your juicer sparkling clean and be rewarded with many years of excellent service. At the time when you acquire your juicer, ask for instructions on how to operate and maintain the machine. Follow instructions for good maintenance.

NATURE'S MEDICINE CHEST

HOW LIVE FOOD JUICES BECOME "NATURE'S PRESCRIPTION" FOR YOUTHFUL HEALTH

The youth-promoting nutrients in raw plant juices help bring about stimulation of the healing forces within the body. Here is a mini-encyclopedia of common and uncommon ailments and how Nature provides an all-natural "prescription" of plant juices for corrective healing.

COLDS. Squeeze two tablespoons of the juice from a fresh, raw onion. Stir quickly into a cup of hot water. Sip throughout the day. Nutrients in the onion are released through squeezing, coming out of the fibers, and are known for nourishing the network of capillaries that have become broken and rendered the susceptibility to colds and sniffles.

CHRONIC FATIGUE. James J., a rugged truckdriver, found himself dozing off behind the wheel. His problem was that he ate heavily and the high fat content in his body drained off the oxygen-bearing supply of blood from his brain to his digestive system. This made him groggy and easily fatigued. His wife provided a natural antidote. She prepared berry juice in a thermos bottle to give to James J. whenever he pulled in for a rest stop. James J. would drink one glass every few hours and he was able to remain awake *without* the use of an artificial stimulant. The secret? Berry juice is rich in natural carbohydrates which are absorbed more readily when taken in juice form; they reach the brain much faster and thus are able to provide valuable oxygen needed to keep alert and alive! Now, James J. is a berry drinker!

HEARTBURN. In this condition, excess acidity in the stomach has become so severe that the acid rises up the gullet to give a feeling of burning in the heart. Instead of alkaline powders which create a vicious addictive-type cycle, look to plant juices. Squeeze out potato juice! The potato is a prime and powerful source of alkaline ingredients that help dilute the excess acid, weaken its burning, and then help it out of the system. Potato juice is Nature's prescription for heartburn.

GASTRIC UPSET. The juice of the cabbage is known for containing instrinsic factors that stabilize gastric acidity and help maintain a normal and soothing flow.

LIVER DISTRESS. Those who are troubled with excessively fatty foods should, of course, adjust their food program to limit such items. To help nourish the tubules of the liver try radish juice. The radish is a prime source of enzymes and minerals that regenerate delicate liver cells. Combine with carrot juice, rich in Vitamin A that is a cellular building nutrient. One glass at noontime helps fortify your internals viscera against many of the ravages of deterioration.

CONSTIPATION. Soak organic prunes in boiled water. Drink the juice first thing in the morning and last thing at night. The rich potassium source is known to be an anti-aging factor and helps rejuvenate the intestinal canal. It is also known for stimulating peristalsis that is needed to establish regularity. This home-made type of prune juice is exceptionally beneficial to those troubled by irregularity.

SKIN BLEMISHES. Susan E. followed corrective food programs but was still troubled with skin blemishes which included acne, unsightly pores, and scale flakes. She was told that *apricot juice* is noteworthy for skin-cleansing. Apricots are rich in iron as well as Vitamins A and C which form a trio of skin-building nutrients. She prepared apricot juice and in combination with other skin cleansing routines, was able to remedy her situation. But she became discouraged since it did not offer "instant beauty" and she gave up the plant juice program. Her acne became so bad that she required chemotherapy and risks possible scarring. She should have had patience with Nature for a lovely skin.

RHEUMATIC DISTRESS. Many who suffer from arm and leg distress report remarkable relief through intake of large amounts of plant juices, especially apple juices. The apple is rich in malic acid, a substance which is able to promote a healing sensation to internal burning-inflammation.

GALL BLADDER. Combine equal amounts of beet juice and lettuce juice. Beets, in particular, are soothing for their high calcium, potassium, and iron content. They nourish the bloodstream which then carries valuable nutrients to all body organs as well as the gall bladder. *Beet leaves* may also be juiced for their powerful iron content.

NERVE DISORDERS. Feel tense? Try a glass of celery juice. Nutrients in celery help eliminate carbon dioxide that often acts as a nerve irritant. Celery has many minerals needed to soothe the nervous system. Raw celery juice is able to stabilize the body's thermostat and keep you cool and collected.

ACID UPSET. Jonathan S. is a much-overworked business executive. For years he was taking all sorts of "stomach pills" to ease recurring acid indigestion. His condition became so bad that he was unable to eat. This weakened him so much that a company doctor who examined him said he might have to be dismissed from the firm. He was heavily in debt with a mortgage, cars, children's education, and could not afford this calamity Desperately, he needed a co-worker's suggestion to eliminate spicy foods and drink up to four glasses of freshly squeezed *lettuce juice* daily. The benefit here is that lettuce is an alkalizer; it also has a rich supply of magnesium which nourishes the nerve system and helps stabilize internal fluidity. He tried lettuce juice, recovered, then slid back to his faulty living habits. He then required long hospitalization for what appeared to be ulcerous conditions. He learned the hard and expensive way that there is no compromise with Nature.

STOMACH PAINS. One time-honored plant juice is that of the pineapple. This fruit contains bromelin which duplicates the action of the hormones of the pancreas. Furthermore, fresh pineapple juice has an enzyme that helps digest food within the abdominal system. It spares the stomach its laborious work and this eases stomach pains. One glass of pineapple juice, one hour after mealtime, is most soothing.

ANEMIA. Build blood by feeding it a high supply of iron. Strawberry juice is a powerhouse of this mineral which works together with calcium phosphorus and the B-complex group. They unite to form a synergistic action that helps nourish the millions of blood cells in the body and correct anemic-like problems. Legend has it that a ripe strawberry helps you look like the fruit of a rose turned inside out—rich and red and youthful.

GENERAL TONIC. Orange juice is rich in its natural sugar content to help provide youthful energy. Raw orange juice helps give tone to the blood vessels by means of sending a stream of oxygen-bearing blood to the brain. Combine with any other fruit juice for a healthfuly and tasty tonic of Nature.

YOUTHFUL STRENGTH. The early Romans worshiped parsley for its strength-building properties. Locked within the tough parsley fibers are powerful vitamins and minerals that should be squeezed out. It reportedly helps the genito-urinary tract, and washes the kidneys and other organs. The juice of the parsley is said to have properties required for oxygen metabolism and also in helping to balance normal adrenal-thyroid hormonal function. Combine parsley juice with the juices of celery or lettuce. Unified, these plant juices help put youth into the body's capillaries and arterial network.

WAKE UP YOUR HIDDEN WELLSPRINGS OF YOUTH. By means of liquid foods—plant juices—you alert and awaken your hidden wellsprings of youth. Plant juices provide your body with the self-healing forces that help to promote the look and feel of healthful youth at any age. Nature meant for you to live long—and youthfully! Let plant juices show you the way!

HIGHLIGHTS OF CHAPTER 1:

1. Liquid foods, also known as plant juices, are known for being able to re-alert your internal wellsprings of youth to give you the look and feel of youth.

2. Ruth W. used raw juices to help turn back the "aging clock."

3. Fresh raw juices help improve assimilation powers, digestive strength, and vitality.

4. Liquid foods have seven benefits that help create the look and feel of youth.

5. Janet Y. followed a raw juice program and defied "heredity" when all said that "illness ran in the family." Raw juices made her healthfully young.

6. Juices provide benefits-plus not found in solid foods.

7. Follow guideline on how and where to prepare your juices.

8. An array of folk healers is made possible by Nature's Medicine Chest using raw live food juices exclusively.

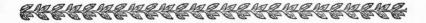

Chapter 2

How Live Food Juices Work to Create

Your Internal "Fountain of Youth"

HELEN Y. was troubled with "sour stomach." She envied folks her own age who could eat to their heart's content with no after-effects. She yearned for luscious steaks, flavorful fish, satisfying casseroles, but had to pass them up because of a recurring problem of what she termed "acid indigestion." She was told that it was an affliction of many "middle-aged" people (even though she was in her 30's) and she had to learn to live with it. This meant that she had to pass up lots of nourishing food and subsist on a meagre, bland and tasteless fare. If she sneaked a juicy slice of roast, she frequently endured severe gas pains and stomach churning gastritis that made her wish she had never tasted any food! Helen Y. rightfully wept because she was denied palatable food because of this affliction.

Impaired Digestion Creates Chronic Fatigue. Helen Y. was denied nourishing food because of so-called "middle-aged digestion" and this had its effect on her general health. Malnutrition meant she could not ingest essential protein foods and she was denied amino acids needed to replenish the entire body. She was unable to properly digest many meats and was deficient in skin and eye building Vitamin A. She could not tolerate bulk foods and had embarrassing constipation together with her gas pains. Helen Y. soon began to look and feel run-down. She had to take increasingly frequent naps. She awoke more tired than when she went to sleep. Little by little, her health was slipping through her fingers.

Chewing Problems Open Way to Liquid Foods. Helen Y's jaw and throat muscles became weak and she felt it difficult to chew foods properly. That was when she started increasing her liquid food intake. A few glasses of fresh vegetable juices helped perk up her health. She found that combinations of certain vegetables helped cool the burning sensation in her chest. Here is one Green Drink that helped correct the severe "bubbling hot gas" sensation that was one core of her problem:

Green Drink for Young Digestion

Juice of 3 freshly scrubbed cucumbers
Juice of fresh green lettuce
Juice of 1 celery bunch
Spoon of lemon juice for flavor

Combine the juices together, stir vigorously, then drink one glass an hour before lunch, another freshly squeezed glass an hour before dinner and a final freshly squeezed glass about one hour before retiring for the night.

Benefit of Green Drink for Young Digestion. A special unique blend of minerals acts upon the alkaline ingredients to help dilute the excess accumulation of gas, rendering it less volatile. Special "binding forces" in the minerals then suck up the acid and help remove it from the system. These vegetAble juices are rich in alkaline ingredients needed to exert a soothing cooling feeling to the digestive organs. They help stabilize a normal and youthful digestive power to promote healthful assimilation of nutrients.

Helen Y. Grows Younger with Green Drink. Because this initial experiment promoted such a feeling of well-being, Helen Y. went on an increased Green Drink program. She would even devote one day to a "juice diet" and subsist entirely on freshly squeezed vegetable juices. In several weeks, her skin had more color, her digestive powers were strengthened, she could eat more wholesomely of good foods, and she felt young again. She looked young, too, because her powers of assimilation meant that extracted nutrients could be put to work to promote the look and feel of youth. She uses the Green Drink for Young Digestion almost daily as Nature's "insurance" for a youthful internal health. She is careful *not* to gorge herself on unnatural foods, and she is grateful to be able to eat and enjoy good food. Nature made her young again!

THE MAGIC YOUTH FEELING OF GREEN DRINKS

Fresh raw vegetables contain a dynamic youth powerhouse of vitamins, minerals, and enzymes that help rebuild and revitalize the digestive system to promote a feeling of youth. Scientists and nutritionists have long confirmed that *you are as young as your digestion.* Improve your digestion and you have the very core of the program designed to give you the look and feel of youth. By means of freshly prepared Green Drinks, you can put a "young feeling" into your digestive system.

SEVEN WAYS IN WHICH GREEN DRINKS PROMOTE YOUTHFUL DIGESTION

Youthful life energy comes from the sun. Green plants know the secret of how to seize this solar vitality and pass it on to man who eats of their leaves. When you touch your body and feel warmth, that warmth and youthful vibrancy has come to you from the sun by way of green plants. The green coloring matter with which Nature endows forests, fields, and gardens, bears a striking resemblance to hemoglobin, the red pigment in human blood. It is as if Nature put "green blood" into her plant foods.

Human blood pigment is a network of carbon, hydrogen, oxygen, and nitrogen atoms, grouped around a single atom of iron. *Plant "blood" pigment* is a similar web of the same atoms except its center is a single atom of youth-building magnesium. You can actually enrich your life and health with plant juices.

Here are the 7 benefits of Green Drinks to promote a youthful digestion and a resultant Look and Feel of Youth of mind and body:

1. *Rich in Enzymes.* Raw plant juices are rich in precious enzymes needed to rebuild your entire system and keep it youthful and healthful.

2. *Vitamin-Mineral Power.* Raw green leaf juices are prime sources of body-building vitamins and organ-nourishing minerals that are easily assimilated. By means of juicing the "locked in" vitamins and minerals are released from the tough fibrous roots, stems, leaves, and branches, and are then sent to speedily perform assimilation in the bloodstream. Here, they are able to provide intimate nourishment of the millions of body cells and tissues, and to help nourish the bloodstream to provide a river of life and youth. Nature-created nutrients in the Green Drink help provide an internal "rebirth" of your vital organs and body processes.

3. *Precious Amino Acids.* Many people who have digestion difficulties are unable to partake of protein foods and deny themselves body-building amino acids. The digestive system must transform eaten protein into amino acids which the body then utilizes. A weak digestion means insufficient metabolization and undigested protein passes out of the system. Green Drinks contain rare and often "hard to get" amino acids which complete the amino acid patterns of so many "incomplete" proteins. Also, Green Drinks are raw and have not had their amino-acid pattern distorted by cooking heat. This benefits the system by saturating it with valuable Nature-prepared

amino acids in the form of a plant juice that require little digestive effort.

4. *Natural Alkaline Balance.* Green leaves in juice form are nearly always alkaline in reaction to the system. Those troubled with gastric distress and addicted to so-called alkalizer medicines, would do well to prepare Green Drinks to help promote a *natural* and *drugless* alkaline balance in the body.

5. *Pure Organic Water.* A freshly prepared Green Drink has up to 90% pure organic water to promote blood enrichment, self-washing, and a refreshing internal comfort. The minerals in the green vegetables are absorbed into this water and sent floating in the bloodstream to wash and replenish the internal network of organs and systems. (Heating converts this to inorganic and lifeless fluid, hence the benefit of fresh *raw* plant juices.)

6. *Self-Cleansing.* The Green Drink also contains bulk or fiber which becomes highly magnetized in its journey through the intestines; this inner-magnetic action draws from the body the used-up tissues and cellular wastes, acting as a broom and self-cleanser. It is this Internal Magnetic Action of the Green Drink that makes it a valuable cleanser to help promote the look and feel of youth. (When greens are cooked, the action is reduced and is said to be more like that of a slimy mop! Again, the emphasis upon health is in the fresh, *uncooked* plant juice.)

7. *Promotes Inner Rejuvenation.* Plant juice stimulates the bone marrow to produce hemoglobin, the red coloring matter of your bloodstream. The Green Drink enables the body to better digest and utilize food, thus increasing resistance to illness and helping to prolong a young feeling. The Green Drink improves and regulates bowel action, strengthens the heart beat, and helps stimulate tissue and cellular repair and growth. It is more beneficial in juice form because the valuable supply of youth-building nutrients are released from the fibrous coils; so, the Green Drink should form a part of your Look and Feel Younger Program. It is a foundation of health.

HOW THE GREEN DRINK WASHES AWAY
ACID INDIGESTION

Andrew E. was a high-strung salesman. Tension made him gobble his food with the consequence that he felt it "back up" in his throat with a burning sensation. He complained that whenever he ate, no matter what he ate, it would cause this acid indigestion.

Eats in Juice Bar and Enjoys Relief. Andrew E. met a customer who invited him to a special juice bar for lunch. He had his first Green Drink, freshly prepared, and exclaimed that he felt a soothing reaction to his system. The Green Drink was made of freshly squeezed cabbage, celery, and spinach. Equal portions of these three vegetables provided soothing minerals that helped weaken the "heat" of the acid produced in the system. Andrew E. felt much better even if he did not close the sale that day.

Improper Eating Habits Create Distress. Andrew E. might have continued on his program of restoring a youthful digestion through the Green Drink except that he was in the habit of bolting down his food, conducting heated arguments during mealtime, imbibing much acid-containing coffee, and eating rich sugar-containing desserts. Sugar is an acid-forming substance and contributes to problems of acid indigestion. Andrew E. consumed more Green Drinks but distress still remained. He had to learn that there is little compromise with Nature. Meet her mid-way and you obtain partial restoration (if any) of health.

Benefit of the Green Drink for Acid Indigestion. Plant extractives that are liberated from tough pulpy fibers during juicing, perform a soothing, tranquilizing and coating action upon the digestive tract. The harsh, volatile and irritated cellular walls are lubricated with these plant juices to help soothe them into relaxation. Plant juices serve to dilute the excess hydrochloric acid that precipitates an attack of indigestion. Often such an attack is like the pain of a heart attack; it is due to a reflux, or backing up, of food into the esophagus from the stomach. Plant juices help soothe the outpouring of volcanic-hot acid and reduce the burning sensation.

Plant juices further coat the esophagus with cooling minerals to help further ease the reaction. *Suggestion:* Mealtime should be a pleasant and cheerful occasion. Tension will only constrict the digestive organs and cause distortion of their functions. Green Drinks are helpful if you are good to your digestion!

YOUR FOUNTAIN OF YOUTH GREEN DRINK

The following Green Drink should be made with a blender. It is a rich source of nutrients that help invigorate the entire digestive organism, thereby promoting effective assimilation of nutrients for a look and feel of youth.

Place one cup fresh pineapple juice in your blender. Add a mixture of several greens (first, wash and remove coarse leaves or woody stems). Push down tightly until blender is about half-full. *Suggestions:* Use mint for its delicious taste; add sprouted seed greens or collards, dandelion, alfalfa, parsley, comfrey, lettuce, spinach. *Small* quantities may be used of watercress, radish or carrot tops or other strong tasting greens.

Blend until finely ground. Add more fresh pineapple juice if desired. Blend for five minutes. Strain, if desired. The benefit of the five minute blending action is to give youth-building enzymes time to release their "green magic" ingredients.

Drink this Fountain of Youth Green Drink twice daily and experience an overall revitalization of your digestive system. The unique benefit here is that this particular drink enters into the powers of *assimilation* within your body. It supercharges the organism with a dynamic look and feel of youth through this regenerated assimilation, the key to vibrant health.

HOW TO USE GREEN LEAVES AS PART OF YOUR "YOUNG AGAIN" PLAN

Adele R. finds there are times when she cannot prepare freshly made juices, but she wants to benefit from plant food in a variety of ways and under all circumstances. Here are some secrets of using green leaves to help promote a "Young Again" feeling:

1. *In large salads.* Adele R. found that her cold hands and cold feet symptoms were relieved through lots of large raw green leaf salads. The benefit here is that minerals in these large raw salads helped to promote a balance of blood circulation through iron absorption and stimulation. Now, her extremities feel comfortably warm and youthful. Large green salads are a "must" for everyday eating.

2. *Green Leaf Tea.* Adele R. had problems with coffee drinking. She liked to drink large amounts of coffee. The excess caffeine so stimulated her that she suffered recurring bouts of insomnia. She looked wan and haggard. She decided to use green leaves for tea! She would steep the leaves in a large teapot or kettle. She would always use mint. She would pour boiling water over the leaves in the kettle and let them sit in a warm place for 20 minutes. She would add a little lemon or honey for flavor and sip slowly. This Green Leaf Tea served as a satisfactory substitute for coffee and was free from the acid-forming effects of drug-like caffeine! It also exerted a warm and tranquil digestive feeling that enabled her to enjoy healthful sleep and a refreshing look of youth.

3. Raw greens may be chopped finely and added to soups or sauces as they are sent to the table. Adele R. would use raw chopped greens to garnish omelets, steamed vegetables, or cooked vegetables.

4. For tough, fibrous vegetables that are healthful but difficult to chew, Adele R. tenderizes them at the lowest possible temperature with a little bit of vegetable oil. This diminishes the highly perishable enzymes which are destroyed by heat, but this low-temperature tenderizing *for the least possible time,* helps release large quantities of other nutrients in the leaves. This facilitates chewing and also releases these nutrients in the digestive tract, when otherwise they might remain locked in the tough fibrous woody stems.

Adele R. now looks the part of a young and healthful hostess and has even aroused the envy of others who scoff at green foods and continue to grow older through their neglect of Nature.

WHY ROOM TEMPERATURE JUICES CREATE DIGESTIVE POWER

If there is to be one proper temperature for juices, it should be room temperature. A comfortably cool juice is soothing and healing. A comfortably warm juice helps promote a more favorable digestion.

Temperature Extremes Inhibit Digestive Function. Very cold or ice-cold juices decrease or halt the flow of digestive enzymes and create impaired digestion. Very hot or volatile hot juices increase a sudden flow of digestive enzymes which often leads to stomach upset. Avoid temperature extremes in consuming your juices.

Iced Juices May "Freeze" Digestion. If juices are made ice cold and consumed with ice cubes, the effect may cause an increased frequency of peristaltic waves so that contractions may even lead to diarrhea. The colder the beverage, the greater the rate of gastric evacuation. Summer diarrhea may be due partly to the ice cold drinks which effect too rapid evacuation of gastric contents not effectively prepared for assimilation because of the "freeze-cold" depression in digestive secretions. It is healthful to avoid temperature extremes of any beverages.

Room Temperature Juices Create Digestive Tonus. Juices consumed at a comfortable natural temperature help increase internal digestive tonus and a normal sphincter muscular contraction. Digestive enzymes are neither scorched nor frozen and are able to send nutrients throughout the body in a comfortably warm environment.

Prepare Juice Immediately After Removing Plants from Refrigerator. To obtain a comfortable temperature, squeeze juices immediately after the fruits and vegetables are removed from the refrigerator and are still cold. This will give you cool juices that are just right for digestive tonus.

HOW GREEN DRINKS PROMOTE "FEEL YOUNG DIGESTIVE POWER"

Roger T. found himself eased out of a comfortable office manager's position because the company decided it was time for him to retire. Roger T. had taken more "sick leave" than in preceding years. Roger T. was getting more easily fatigued. All this when he was in his late 50's which meant he should have had better years ahead of him. But his chronic allergic distress coupled with a severe case of gastritis left him weak and spent. So his superiors eased him into retirement at a time when he needed the money to pay off his mortgage and also save for a much anticipated worldwide trip with his wife. A company doctor told him that he might find relief through a special prescribed medication that would perform the same benefits as minerals in green vegetables!

Roger Looks to Vegetable Healing. It occurred to Roger that if minerals in vegetables could soothe his gastritis, perhaps it was wiser to obtain them from plant juices than chemical juices at a pharmacy. He started drinking copious amounts of fresh raw plant juices and obtained considerable relief from his stomach churning distress. But Roger's problem was that he liked fat-coated fried foods and this created digestive upset. Only when he gave them up in favor of healthfully broiled meats, could he enjoy reasonable freedom from digestive weakness.

Alfalfa Juice Promotes "Feel Young Digestive Power." At a health store, Roger obtained alfalfa seeds. He would make a tea out of the seeds and use the juice, so to speak, for healing. Alfalfa juice (or tea) was originally called "green gold" for its healing powers. It is rich in alkali-forming nutrients. It is said to have double the protein supply of wheat and corn grains. The unique youth-building properties of this "green gold" lie in its essential amino acids such as arginine, lysine, and threonine. These serve to stabilize the internal mechanisms that promote healthful digestion. Roger T. began his recovery from a lifetime of digestive weakness, obtained another position and was even able to "fib" about his age since he looked much younger again. He drinks two glasses of Green Juices every single day as "youth insurance."

THE FOUNTAIN OF YOUTH POWER IN GREEN DRINKS. Your body and your mind live in a constant state of movement. Vitamins, minerals, enzymes, and amino acids found in the Green Drink enter into the bloodstream. This powerhouse exerts a "Fountain of Youth" that keeps each body cell in a state of dynamic equilibrium, endlessly changing each trillionth of a second to nourish, regenerate, and rejuvenate your digestive system.

How Green Drinks Promote a Youth-Creating Homeostasis.
its power to create the wn as *homeostasis,* or a our body seeks to sustain ilizing the nutrients given ices or the Green Drinks. is that the Green Drinks ain these trillions of body elp thwart and correct the digestion comes from a t is invigorated with fresh through natural Green ealthful digestive youth.

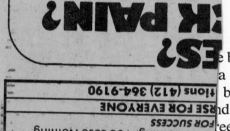

e by using Green Drinks to a young feeling. benefits in promoting a d Feel of Youth. een Drinks.

4. A Fountain of Youth Green Drink promotes digestive assimilation.
5. Adele R.'s program of plant juices helped make her "grow younger."

6. Room temperature juices boost digestive tonus.

7. Roger T.'s Alfalfa Juice or "green gold" drink promoted homeostasis or the "young feel" of his digestive system. All natural!

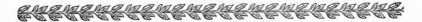

Chapter 3

Healthful Elixirs to Help Put

Youthful Glamour into Your Skin

YOU can drink your way to a younger looking complexion! A nutritiously healthful skin creates more than just the look and feel of youth. It helps promote overall physical rejuvenation. Healthful elixirs in special combinations promote an enrichment of the cellular tissues beneath the skin, thereby nourishing this body envelope so that it can help keep you well. When nutrients and substances in healthful elixirs nourish the skin, the overall benefits include:

1. *Protection Against Aging.* A well-nourished skin helps ward off microbes and bacteria, preventing their entrance into the body where they promote the aging processes. Nutrients in elixirs and live food juices help strengthen the skin so that it can resist external chemical ravages, throw off unwanted radioactivity, and shield against noxious gases. A healthy skin is able to cover the bones, muscles and other body structures and keep you looking and feeling young.

45

2. *Regulates Body Temperature.* Live food juices are rich in minerals that nourish the nerve endings of the skin and help maintain a pleasing body temperature. Live food juices are especially skin-beneficial in that they require relaxed digestive action and are speedily assimilated. This means that heat generated inside the body by the *easy* digestion of live food juices will produce a self-regulating body temperature and a calm metabolism. The bloodstream carries this heat to the skin and the skin dissipates it back into the atmosphere. Live food juices are gentle to this temperature-regulating process and help keep you comfortably cool or warm as the situation warrants.

3. *Youthful Nerve Sensation.* The so-called "age twitches" or excessively nervous skin sensitivity need not occur with the presence of nutrients in live food juices. A rich supply of minerals in live food juices helps nourish the nerve endings (known as *pacinian corpuscles*) located beneath the skin surface. These minerals enable such nerve endings to transport sensations of heat, cold, and pressures. Enzymes in live food juices are generators in that they help send messages from these skin nerve endings to the brain and back to controlling muscles. Vitamins and amino acids in juices then help nourish the blood vessels that relax the nervous condition of "goose pimples" caused by nutrient-starved constricted blood vessels. Feed your vessels healthful nutrients in live food juices and they become youthfully healthy.

4. *Self-Cleansing Benefit.* Nutrients in live food juices promote the process of secretion or self-cleansing. The nutrients in live juices nourish the sebaceous glands which are found deep in the skin's inner layers. This sets up an inner working mechanism by which the well-nourished bloodstream provides the materials to the sebaceous glands to help "suck up" wastes to be cast off through skin pores in the form of perspiration. Live juices are brimming with the nutrients that the bloodstream needs to use for "magnetic" action through the sebaceous glands. Without sufficient nutrients, wastes cannot be cast off and the resultant condition may be wrinkles, unsightly blemishes, so-called "age spots," acne, and

premature aging skin. Live food juices may well be the key to skin youth.

5. *Youthful Acid Mantle.* A healthful skin that looks and feels young to the touch is one that has an acid mantle. This is made possible by emphasizing two special nutrients which are found in food juices: *amino acids* and *unsaturated fatty acids*. In combination, these two nutrients will help promote a healthful acid mantle that wards off infectious bacteria and helps promote the look and feel of a young skin.

BEAUTY FARM SECRET OF SKIN FOOD. A famous beauty farm, visited by women of royalty, society, and theatre, is aware of the powers of live food juices to promote an acid mantle to the skin. Here is their Beauty Farm Skin Food beverage, consumed by patrons three times daily:

> 3 tablespoons peanut oil
> 3 tablespoons apple cider vinegar
> 1/2 cup lettuce juice
> 1/2 cup carrot juice
> Honey to taste

Mix all ingredients together until totally assimilated. Drink three times daily. The unique benefit to the skin here is that the blending of the amino acids and unsaturated fatty acids together with the "magnetic" action of the vitamins and minerals, helps nourish the delicate skin cells and also maintain a normal and healthful *hydrogen ion* state. The key to a normal acid mantle of look-feel young skin is in the balance of the hydrogen ion state known as the pH system or the so-called acid level of the skin. The nutrients in the Beauty Farm Skin Food beverage work together to perform this *hydrogen ion* state and create a youthful pH balance. Now you can prepare this expensive beauty farm's formula right in your own home for a modest cost and a few moments of time.

6. *Skin-Breathing for Health.* The skin may not have lungs, but it does breathe by taking in oxygen and casting off carbon dioxide. To help this skin-breathing function, there is a need for adequate vitamins, minerals and enzymes that can work speedily to promote this function. Live food juices contain

living nutrients prepared by Nature and help promote this vital skin-breathing process.

HOW FOOD JUICES CAN MOISTURIZE YOUR SKIN TO GLOWING YOUTHFULNESS

Linda R. was a fashion consultant who spent a big part of her budget for the right clothes. She had to look the picture of fashion in order to sell styles to others. Her problem was that while her clothes in the latest style gave the appearance of youth, her skin looked dry, had crease lines that were developing into wrinkles and showed signs of starting to sag. She wore more costly clothes in the hopes the reflection on her skin would create a youthful glow. She even spent much money on expensive cosmetics which helped hide some of the dry skin wrinkles, but did not correct the cause—lack of sufficient internal moisture.

Salesgirl Suggests Juices. Linda R. changed cosmetics and bought all-natural makeup at a natural foods outlet. She chatted with the salesgirl who had a "blooming red rose" complexion. The salesgirl said that cosmetics helped enhance and color the complexion, but it could not correct the cause of aging and scaliness. That, said the salesgirl, had to be corrected by improving the "moisture supply" beneath the surface. Where to obtain moisture? Through fresh living food juices. The salesgirl urged Linda to try a special home recipe that worked for herself.

Skin Moisturizing Food Tonic. Mix equal portions of seasonal berry juice, blend with one-half cup of apricot juice, season with honey. Drink one glass before breakfast, another glass during lunchtime, a third glass before the evening meal.

Unique benefits: The unusual benefits lie in the rich mineral power. These live food juices are especially rich in sulphur and copper. This latter mineral, copper, unites with iron, and helps manufacture hemoglobin, the oxygen-carrying ingredient in the red blood cells. The Skin Moisturizing Food Tonic then works to activate the tiny "moisture reservoirs" that lie deep beneath the surface of the skin to promote a natural oil that helps lubricate the skin cells and tissues. The Skin Moisturizing Food Tonic thereby promotes a naturally lubricated skin that helps protect against wrinkling and so-called "age spots."

Linda R. Looks Younger. Linda R. tried this special live food tonic and in a week or two, did have a younger looking complexion. But her success was short-lived. She may have nourished her skin and body with natural live food juices, but she contradicted Nature by heavy smoking, alcoholic drinks, endless cups of corrosion-creating coffee, not to mention bleached white foods and artificial additive-containing foods. These created internal havoc, dried out the "moisture reservoirs" and made Linda look older than before. She gave up the alliance with Nature and just applied more and more makeup. Unhappily, she continued to look and grow older. This could have been avoided if she had placed herself in Nature's hands and drunk deep of the wealth in youth-creating live food juices.

THE AGELESS SKIN YOUTH OF THE GRECIANS

Men and women in the Mediterranean are known for having young-looking complexions. The Grecians, in particular, share honors with the Italians for having smooth, wrinkle-free skin and glossy shiny hair. The secret here lies in the power of *oils* that help promote a skin that is youthfully delightful to the eye and touch.

How Oils Help Promote Youthful Skin. The unsaturated fatty acids in vegetable and seed oils promote production of lubricating substances in the tiny oil and moisture "wells" that are located within the skin. These vegetable and seed oils help the moisture "wells" establish a delicate balance by regulating the amount of lubrication to help create a soft, young, and well-nourished "alive" looking skin.

Favorite Oils: Amongst the favorite oils that help create this inner moisture are those made from the almond, apricot kernel, avocado, cocoanut, corn, cottonseed, olive, peanut, safflower, sesame, soybean, sunflower, walnut, and wheat germ. You may use these oils singly or in a combination.

How to Use Oils: Use on fresh raw vegetable salads. Take two tablespoons with a glass of freshly squeezed vegetable juice. Use oils in cooking processes but heating may cause depletion of essential amino acids and minerals, so it is wise to use sparingly. The maximum skin benefit from oils is in their natural state with a salad or mixed with a vegetable juice.

GREEK BEAUTY NIGHT OIL PROGRAM. A well-known fashion model who is in her late 30's, but looks in her late 'teens, takes exceptional care of her skin with a special program. Katina E. has followed a time-honored Mediterranean folk secret that dates back to when the peoples of the Aegean Sea boasted beauty the world over. Katina E. will take four tablespoons of any available seed oil, together with one tablespoon of apple cider vinegar, and mix it all together in a cup of vegetable juice.

She drinks this about one hour before going off to sleep. It is this simple yet amazingly effective Greek folk secret that may be responsible for her smooth-as-a-statue skin that glows with the bursting sunshine of dawn over the Mediterranean.

Oil Works While You Sleep. Katina E. has discovered that the seed oil taken before bedtime is able to work while you sleep. During sleep when the body is at rest, the unsaturated fatty acids together with the potassium of the apple cider vinegar, join with the minerals and enzymes in the vegetable juice. This combination creates an isotonic action which is programmed by Nature to transport skin-improving fluids directly to the cells and tissues where they are most needed.

Oil Boosts Skin Health. Being amazingly compatible with the natural liquids of the skin, this Greek Beauty Night Oil Program with its moist oil content, unites with existing supplies of natural oils. *Special benefit:* It helps regenerate and boost the sluggish cellular levels so that the skin is encouraged to self-stimulate its own equilibrium and help provide natural nourishment to these tiny "moisture reservoirs" which rule the skin's health and youthful beauty. All this in natural live juices—that is, the juices of Nature's seeds and vegetables and fruits in a time-honored folk remedy. Small wonder that Katina E. looks decades younger—without the need of makeup. Nature helps give her the look and feel of youth by alerting the inner moisture wells and springs of lubrication.

AUSTRIAN BEAUTY SALON AND THE SKIN OIL PROGRAM

Many European and American women come to a famous Austrian beauty salon for help with their skin problems. The cosmetologists here have had remarkable success in rejuvenating the "aging" skin of women (and men, too!) by emphasizing the need for replenishing the sluggish oil-producing glands beneath the skin surface. In particular, they urge their customers to eliminate artificial foods from their diets, and emphasize fresh live food juice with its rich supply of enzymes and minerals. They also have prepared this unique mayonnaise that can be used with salads as a dressing, or it can be put in a cup and actually eaten with a spoon, by itself! This particular mayonnaise contains the ingredients that are needed by the skin to stimulate sluggish glands to produce much needed oils. Here is the Austrian Beauty Salon's Skin Food Mayonnaise:

> 2 fresh egg yolks
> $1/2$ cup sunflower oil
> $1/2$ cup sesame oil
> 1 tablespoon wheat germ oil
> 1 tablespoon apple cider vinegar

Mix the oils in a measuring cup. Put fresh egg yolks in a cold bowl and beat. Add oil, slowly at first; beat with a rotary beater. Add more oil gradually. As the mixture thickens, add the apple cider vinegar. Put in a cup and eat slowly with a spoon. *Or,* use as a salad dressing.

Benefits of Austrian Beauty Salon's Skin Food Mayonnaise: The fresh egg yolks supply lecithin, a remarkable oil-producing skin softener and Vitamin A, a nutrient that helps nourish skin tissues. The apple cider vinegar is mildly acid and helps promote the hydrogen ion state for a normal pH skin acidity. The oils are powerful sources of unsaturated fatty acids that help sustain the delicate balance of moisture required for the dew-fresh appearance of a youthful complexion. This Austrian Skin Food helps provide a steady flow of rich moist oil, *beneath* the surface of the skin, and enables the skin to maintain resilience and a fine-grained texture. It promotes a lovely smoothness and eases the tendency of the skin to dry out and endure age spots. Skin youth must come from *within,* and oils are able to promote a complexion that is soft, smooth and blooming with youth.

THE FRUIT THAT GIVES YOU A
GOLDEN SKIN GLOW

Raymond T. worked outdoors in inclement weather. He was constantly catching cold. His wife knew that lots of fresh fruit juices would provide a supply of Vitamin C that would help build resistance to colds and winter ailments. So she would give him a thermos container with freshly prepared fruit juice. Raymond T. found that he was less susceptible to colds if he would drink at least one quart of fresh fruit juice a day. But he noted another benefit.

Raymond's Skin Looks Younger. His skin, subjected to harsh climatic elements and atmospheric pollution and smog, now lost its sickish pallor. It began to glow and look healthfully young. The color was enriched and the flabbiness was made firm. He did not think it had anything to do with his raw juice program. When warm weather came and there was no risk of cold-catching, he discontinued the thermos of the fruit juice. He did not catch cold again since it was summertime, but his complexion began to grow waxen, develop folds and look aged. His wife deduced that it must have been the fruit juice that had produced his healthy skin before so she gave him a daily thermos. However, in her area of the country, certain citrus fruits were out of season. How to prepare a quart? She mixed orange juice with lemon juice, going heavy on the lemon juice because lemons were in abundance and at low cost. Again, Raymond's skin improved and he reflected the glow of youth.

Raymond's Wife Shares in Nature's Skin Food. Envious, his wife started taking half-and-half mixtures of any available fruit juice and lemon juice. She felt her skin growing softer and looking better. She made fruit juice a daily fare; Raymond, meanwhile, turned it down because he said it was for women only! So his wife enjoyed a youthful skin while Raymond denied Nature and denied himself the look and feel of youth.

HOW LEMON JUICE PROMOTES SKIN HEALTH. Lemons are a prime source of Vitamin C. This nutrient promotes the health of the skin's connective tissues (the tissues which bind all the individual cells together, compose cartilage, veins, and ligaments). As the red blood cells carry oxygen to each individual body cell, so Vitamin C from lemon juice carries hydrogen, another ingredient needed for metabolism and nourishment of the skin tissues. The lemon juice's Vitamin C causes the proper absorption of iron in the body to help nourish the skin tissues. Lemons may well hold the secret of the look and feel of youthful skin.

Lemon Juice Promotes Skin Rejuvenation. Nutrients in lemon juice help promote the complete and natural rhythm of skin tissue renewal and are able to bring out the natural bloom of youthful health.

Lemon Juice Creates Skin Birth. The nutrients in lemon juice are assimilated into the bloodstream and a unique skin-birth cycle begins. The nutrients help the skin in its own capacity to shed and replace the outermost layer of closely-locked cellular scales of which it is made. The clinging of destroyed cells to the skin inhibits healthy functioning; this is one prime cause of premature aging on the skin. Lemon juice with its released enzymes helps to tone the skin, to invigorate it. Enzymes in the lemon juice work to stimulate Nature's efforts to exert a steady production of new cell creation. This works to promote a fresh and smooth skin quality.

Lemon Juice Creates Flaking Process. Vitamin C is released to join with enzymes to help the natural "flaking" process of discarded and unnecessary skin cells. This action causes a gentle coaxing away of old, clinging, aging particles of "crepe skin" and enables new cells to take their place to create a healthy new skin tonus.

Lemon Juice Whips Up Skin Metabolism. Nutrients in lemon juice work to stimulate and whip up skin metabolism; this leads to a relaxation of tense face and neck muscles, awakening the skin to youthful life. Furthermore, the action of the nutrients in lemon juice encourages the "melting out" of clogging grime and wastes that contribute to blemishes and aging complexion. One unique benefit of enzyme-rich lemon juice: *the enzymes help improve the vital acid-alkali balance on the skin which makes all the difference between an aging and a youthful complexion.*

Through means of live food juices, proper nourishment is transported constantly through the bloodstream to the tiny vessels of the dermis so that your skin will remain healthy, clear and free from unnecessary blemishes.

LEMON JUICE SKIN COCKTAIL. Because the lemon juice is rather tart, it is wise to use just several tablespoons together with another fresh fruit juice. Mix and (if desired) add one egg yolk that is beaten in a blender for thorough assimilation. This gives you valuable vitamins, minerals, enzymes, and unsaturated fatty acids to help promote a youthful looking skin.

HOW TO DRINK A "BEAUTY BREAKFAST"

Breakfast is, indeed, the most important meal of the day. Yet Arnold E., who was either too sleepy or too sluggish in the wee hours of the morning, was a breakfast skipper. It had its effect on his health. He was frequently sleepy by mid-morning, and had to take an early lunch to help provide needed nourishment and energy. But Arnold E. had another problem.

Looks Sickish and Has "Crepe-Like" Face. A nutritional

deficiency took its toll of his skin which developed unsightly "accordion folds" and gave him a "crepe-like" complexion. Even his lips were pale; the corners of his mouth were cracked. His tongue was cracked and inflamed. He developed serious itching problems. His skin began to age! Improper food was taking its toll.

How Arnold E. Could Drink His Breakfast and Help Rejuvenate His Skin and Health. Because he was always in a hurry, he felt that if he had to eat breakfast, he might try one of the instant types. It might be mentioned that a company physician examined the chronically ill Arnold and suggested that he take a liquid breakfast if he had neither time nor appetite. However, the prepared liquid packaged breakfasts were so loaded with preservatives, Arnold E. shunned them. A shopper in a large store told him how his wife prepared a healthful breakfast that provided pep, vigor, and good skin tonus. Arnold tried it. Now he could drink his breakfast. Here is the special *Beauty Breakfast:*

> Juice of three fresh oranges *or* pineapple juice
> 4 tablespoons natural raw wheat germ
> 1 teaspoon brewer's yeast
> 1 tablespoon soya powder
> 1 banana
> Honey to taste
> 1 teaspoon blackstrap molasses
> 1 teaspoon whey powder
> 4 sliced apricots (sun-dried, organic variety)

All of the ingredients were placed in a blender and set a-whirring for five minutes. Then Arnold would sip it slowly, enjoying every drop of Nature's healthful beverage—one big glass each morning.

Skin Building Benefits of Beauty Breakfast: The fruit juice was rich in skin-nourishing Vitamin C. The yeast had a strong supply of the B-complex vitamins which rejuvenate the nervous system. The soya powder was a powerhouse of amino acids that regenerate tissues and cells. The molasses, honey, banana, and apricots were rich in minerals which combined with the other elements to exert a powerful enzymatic action in natural restoration of healthful powers. In combination, the Beauty Breakfast worked to give Arnold E. the pep, vigor, and the "Young Again" skin he deserved. Nature promoted this natural healing and helped give Arnold E. a "second chance" on youth. He looked young and he felt young.

Live Food Elixirs Promote Youthful Skin Glamour. The moisture-craving cells and tissues of the skin require liquids to satisfy their thirst. Give them live food elixirs to drink and they will reward you with a healthful skin that you will love to touch!

SUMMATION:

1. Live food juices and elixirs produce five benefits to a healthy skin.

2. The Beauty Farm Skin Food maintains a healthful hydrogen ion state of skin youth.

3. Live food elixirs help moisturize the skin. The Skin Moisturizing Food Tonic helped Linda R. inhibit aging conditions.

4. The peoples of the Mediterranean used oils to maintain youthful skin tonus.

5. The Greek Beauty Night Oil Program helps lubricate skin cells while you sleep! You awaken with a youthful skin.

6. A special Austrian Beauty Salon's Skin Food Mayonnaise helps promote softening and replenishment of "tired" tissues.

7. Lemons reputedly hold the secret elixir for skin regeneration.

8. A special Beauty Breakfast (for men and women alike) helps promote an overall feeling of a youthful skin. It serves as the foundation for your Look and Feel Young Program.

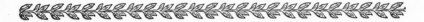

Chapter 4

How Folk Potions May Help Stimulate

Hair Growth on the Head

IF there is one part of your body that is part of the image of youth, it is your hair! If your hairline is receding, or if your hair is thinning even at a mature age, it indicates that something has gone awry with your metabolic system and corrective measures should be taken.

HOW LIQUID FOODS MAY CORRECT HAIR DISTRESS. Hair is constructed of the same kind of tissue as the outer layer of skin, or epidermis, and it requires nourishment in a similar manner. Hair grows in a tiny indentation in the skin, called a follicle, at the base of which is tissue containing blood vessels which supply food to the hair. The purpose here is to give natural food to the tissues that contain blood vessels. In that manner, you may help nourish your scalp. Some people lose hair at an early age; others lose hair at a later age. Many others never lose their hair! True, some factors of heredity are involved but metabolism is *not* an inherited factor. And since hair growth is related to metabolism, it holds true that proper nutrition may well conquer the problem of hair loss.

Liquid foods are especially beneficial because they have easily assimilated nutrients that go to work speedily as soon as they are introduced to the system. These enzymes and nutrients should be able to feed the hair bulb and help control your hair health.

THE FOOD PROGRAM TO ENCOURAGE HAIR HEALTH

Many investigators have related hair health to proper food practices. Here is a special Food Program to Encourage Hair Health that serves as the foundation of your plans:

1. *Germinating Foods Promote Follicle Youth.* Germinating foods are non-processed edibles such as seeds, nuts, grains, fertile eggs, raw butter, non-pasteurized milk, fresh fruits and vegetables. The emphasis is on *untouched by contamination* foods. This means you should eliminate foods that have been salted, processed, pre-heated, sweetened, preserved, dehydrated, pre-cooked, etc. Germinating foods provide the "germ" to feed enzymes to your follicles to help promote a youthful hair growing environment.

2. *Two Vitamins Promote Healthy Metabolism.* It is essential to include Vitamins B and E because they help strengthen nerve endings, stimulate oxidation, help remove toxic wastes, and refresh the metabolic system. These vitamins are found in yeast, wheat germ, wheat germ oil, desiccated liver, sunflower seeds, pumpkin seeds and—raw fruits and vegetables. These are "must" foods in your hair growing program.

3. *A Clean Scalp is a Healthy Scalp.* With so much pollution and fallout, the hair is a catch basin for refuse and dirt. Cleanliness is essential. Use a natural shampoo, brush daily, avoid harsh chemical tonics and hair sprays. Well-brushed hair that is healthy will form its own natural style on the head.

4. *Drink Your Way to a Healthy Scalp.* Fresh liquid juices are rich in the nutrients needed by your scalp. Drink fresh juices daily.

HOW LIQUID FOODS HELP PROMOTE SCALP ENERGY FOR HAIR GROWTH

Leonard R. noticed his thinning hair. He had tried one patent medicine after another, ran the gamut of tonics and chemical lotions which worsened his hair health and caused increasing loss.

Desperate and embarrassed (he was only 36 and being called unflattering names by more generously endowed "friends"), he started researching everything he could on the subject of hair growth. He then came up with research on folk potions and suggestions on how the scalp could be "energized" to help grow hair. Here is one reported Hair-Growing Potion that he tried:

1. Put six tablespoonfuls of whole milk into a small screw-top jar or blender. Milk should be raw—preferably certified. Or, substitute with soya bean milk.

2. Add one tablespoon of cold-pressed wheat germ oil. Cover and shake or blend up to 15 seconds.

3. Drink this Hair Growing Potion promptly.

4. Most favorable time is about a half hour before breakfast *or* four hours after the evening meal.

Added benefit: Drink this Hair Growing Potion on an empty stomach so that the ingested nutrients can be metabolized without the interference of other substances.

Results: Leonard R. was *not* able to restore lost hair, but after six weeks of this program, augmented with an all-natural food program, he was able to halt hair loss. His own hair looked thicker, better and it remained—even for years after the hair of his friends fell out. Leonard R. continues with this Hair Growing Potion. It's all natural!

How Hair-Growing Potion Helps Energize the Scalp. Looking at the scalp, we note it is more generously supplied with hair follicles than any other part of the body. A hair follicle is a tiny pocket pushing into the skin from the surface. Its bottom has a cellular cluster called the *matrix* from which hair grows. This matrix produces about 1/100 of an inch of hair every day.

Requires Energy. The secret here is that the matrix must have energy to produce this amount of hair. This energy is taken from the body's metabolism. Denied this very large energy supply, the matrix cannot summon sufficient power to produce this hair growth and there is either deficiency, decline, or loss.

Potion Provides Energy. The ingredients in the preceding Hair Growing Cocktail worked to send a stream of energy-producing vitality by means of the unsaturated fatty acids in the milk. This combination exerted a boost that fed the matrix through the bloodstream and regenerated the follicle. To help stimulate hair growth, energize your scalp with the Hair Growing Potion.

HOW TO NOURISH YOUR SCALP TO
BETTER HAIR HEALTH

Irma T. is a corporation stenographer. She spends days on end in board room meetings, taking down notes, unable to obtain fresh air, subjecting her body and her scalp to incessant amounts of clouds of thick cigar smoke. Yet Irma T. has found that if she brushes her hair, observes hygienic rules of cleanliness, improves her food program and drinks a special Hair Health Juice, she has a nourished scalp and healthy hair.

Here is Irma T.'s special Hair Health Juice: To one cup of skimmed milk, add one tablespoon of pure gelatin, one teaspoon of sesame oil, one teaspoon of honey or any fruit juice flavor. Mix together in a blender or just stir vigorously. Drink it in the morning and in the evening.

Benefit of Health Hair Juice. Irma T. nourishes her scalp with this live food juice. The gelatin is a power-packed source of hair-growing protein which doubles and whips up the mineral power of the milk. This Hair Health Juice contains nerve health B-complex and calcium. The *special benefit-plus* here is in the rich supply of unsaturated fatty acids in the sesame oil which anoint the follicles and help combat dryness, dandruff, and eventual hair loss. This combination alerts Irma's body, her scalp and the hair-growing processes so she can have a healthy head of hair even though she subjects it to abuse from indoor smoke-grimed living.

Basic Food Program: Irma T., in addition, corrects her food program. She knows that sweet and fatty foods have a bad effect on the sebaceous glands as well as the hair follicles, so she omits them. She eats foods that are high in protein such as lean meat, fish, eggs, cottage cheese, and soybeans; she also drinks lots of fresh fruit and vegetable juices. She has a young skin, a young head of hair—and a young attitude! Nature helped her!

HOW SEED JUICE HELPS INVIGORATE SCALP

A folk program calls for preparing special *Hair Health Seed Juice,* as follows:

Place a quarter cup of unsprayed, organically-grown seeds in a quart-size jar. Cover with a square of double thickness cheesecloth. Fasten with a rubber band. Fill the jar half full with water. Let stand overnight.

Next morning: drain off this water and use it as a Seed Juice beverage by itself, or combine with a little vegetable juice and a spoon of honey.

Sprout Seeds: Now, rinse the seeds with fresh water. Pour off the rinse. Set the jar inverted (but slightly tipped) so that any remaining water may drain off. A good site for sprouting would be a slightly warm and dark cupboard. Now, let the jar remain.

How to Rinse: Twice each day (morning and night) give the seeds a fresh-water rinse, replace in the same inverted position.

Several Days Later: The seeds will have tiny sprouts. You may eat these sprouts in a salad or by themselves.

Benefits of Seed Juice and Seed Sprouts for Scalp Nourishment: Sprouting endows seeds and grains with Vitamin C and multiplies their vitamin, mineral and enzyme values. These nutrients are required by "weak" sites of your body, especially the scalp where hair loss indicates an error or deficiency in metabolism. The juice and the sprouts are powerful supplies of *germinating* nutrients that help nourish the scalp and create a good hair growing environment.

Beneficial Seeds to Use: Good seeds for sprouting may be alfalfa, lentils, mung beans, garbanzas, wheat, peas, radishes, kale, or turnips. Ask at any organic seed outlet or health store for available seeds.

Drink and Eat Daily. It is wise to drink the Seed Juice daily. It is also healthful to use the seed sprouts daily with salads or for munching. Your weakened metabolism as evidenced by poor hair health indicates the need for much seed juice.

A VITAMIN HAIR-GROWING COCKTAIL

Vitamin E is unique in that it may help nourish the hair bulb and improve the hair growth.

It is medically known that the biological activity of the hair bulb depends upon the maintenance of a high level of energy production in the cells. This depends upon an available supply of glucose and oxygen. Vitamin E protects the body's store of oxygen and it is believed that the effect of extra Vitamin E on the hair bulb, introduced through liquid foods, will help increase hair growth.

How Vitamin E Provides Oxygen to Hair Bulb. Vitamin E performs a known youth-giving function of oxygen conservation within the body. It is Nature's own anti-oxidant. It helps decrease the oxygen requirement of muscle by as much as 43 per cent, and helps promote blood to all body parts, including the "choked" scalp. Sufficient oxygen is vital to help rejuvenate the scalp and promote hair health.

Make Your Own *Vitamin Hair Growing Cocktail:*

> $1/4$ cup wheat germ oil (cold-pressed)
> $1/4$ cup soybean oil
> 4 tablespoons apple cider vinegar
> $1/2$ cup fresh vegetable oil

Mix vigorously and eat with a spoon. Slowly sip and swallow. One such cocktail a day will provide much oxygen-producing

Vitamin E that reportedly helps create scalp health for favorable hair invigoration.

Why The Avocado is A Good Hair-Growth Vitamin Source. It has been noted that Vitamin E is better assimilated into the body if you select a plant food that is non-cellulose. The avocado is said to be without rival in providing more absorption of Vitamin E in the body than other foods. Of course, wheat germ oil is the prime source and has the highest potency of Vitamin E. It might be wise to squeeze several tablespoons of avocado oil onto your salads daily. Also, include the Vitamin Hair Growing Cocktail (a powerhouse of Vitamin E and minerals) in your daily corrective hair scalp program. This cocktail sends a stream of Vitamin E into the body to protect the store of oxygen and to nourish the hair bulb, among other necessary functions.

EDNA J. GROWS "HEALTHY HAIR" BY FEEDING HER THYROID GLAND

Edna J. was so embarrassed by her increasing hair loss, not to mention the dull "mop-like" look her hair had, that she became nervous and high-strung. She wore hats as often as possible, but this did not correct the cause of her loss.

Thirsty Thyroid Drinks Its Way to Healthy Hair. Edna's sister alerted her to an inactive thyroid. In the sister's condition, a weak thyroid gland made her thin, nervous, high-strung, and slow moving. She suggested Edna try some good health tonics that would promote a youthful thyroid and also correct the condition of poor hair health. Here is the Thyroid Elixir that helped Edna J.:

> $1/2$ cup unsweetened gelatin powder
> 2 tablespoons brewer's yeast
> $1/2$ cup freshly squeezed orange juice

She would drink this Thyroid Elixir thrice daily. In two weeks, Edna J. was much improved and her health showed in better looking hair.

Sister Errs in Her Thyroid Elixir. Edna's sister was so enthused by the visible results, she made her own Thyroid Elixir but she neglected to add brewer's yeast and the results were so slight that she gave up in disgust. She neglected her own thyroid weakness until she had to be hospitalized for a nervous breakdown. Why didn't the Thyroid Elixir work for Edna's sister?

Secret: The secret lies in the benefits of the *combined* action of the above three ingredients. The protein in the gelatin powder helped feed the activity of a sluggish thyroid gland by supplying the amino acid *tyrosine* (from which the thyroid hormone is made.) However, tyrosine cannot be utilized without the activation of the B-complex vitamins found in such food as brewer's yeast. Furthermore, thyroxin (the natural hormone of the thyroid that is responsible for hair health) itself becomes inactivated by oxygen if there is a deficiency of Vitamin C found in fresh fruit juice. It is a working together of proteins—B-complex and Vitamin C— that feed a thirsty thyroid and help regulate its hormonal flow to promote overall health—including hair health.

The Thyroid Elixir is beneficial for promoting this triple action upon the thyroid gland which governs health of personality, hormonal system and, of course, the health of the hair!

USE A NATURAL BRISTLE HAIR BRUSH. George R., at age 27, became alarmed over his increasing hair loss. He would try the Thyroid Elixir and also other liquid foods, and follow the natural laws of healthful living, yet he soon developed an almost bald region of a triangular shape on the right side of his head. It steadily increased during the year. Regrowth did not appear.

George R., when questioned, said he would brush his hair twice daily, using a nylon hairbrush. This was a clue to the problem. He was told to use a natural bristle brush at once. (Nylon or synthetic brushes tear out the hair from the roots and shafts.)

Increases Liquid Foods and Corrective Brushing. George R. switched to a natural bristle hair brush. He also increased his intake of natural liquid foods as outlined in this chapter. It took three months and the area was soon covered with strong hair of normal length and appearance. He had relied upon Nature even to the use of a natural bristle brush and his hair health improved.

A SUGAR-FREE PROGRAM HELPS PROMOTE HEALTHY HAIR. Claire T. could not understand why she failed to enjoy a healthy scalp even though she enjoyed a variety of special liquid foods. Under questioning, it was found that she would saturate the beverages with white sugar. This had a negative effect. Claire T. was told to eliminate white sugar from her entire eating program. It took several months until her overall body health was revitalized and the liquid foods promoted the look and feel of youth that was reflected in a head of healthy hair.

Hair-Destroying Power of Sugar. Sugar often replaces protein in the metabolism process. It was found that a deficiency of protein and surplus of sugar may cause decreased pigmentation and atrophy of hair. An acid non-food, white sugar (whether consumed in white powder as a sweetener for beverages, or included in baked and cooked goods, candies, pies, sweet desserts, etc.) has a corrosive and destructive action on the scalp and the delicate papillae of the scalp. Eliminate artificial sweeteners and sugar and give your hair a better chance to grow!

AN OIL RUB ON THE SCALP IS HELPFUL. To help relieve a dry scalp, a vegetable oil rub is helpful. Recommended oils include olive, sesame, peanut, or sunflower, in conjunction with small amounts of solubilized lanolin, such as isopropyl or acetylated lanolin (available at most pharmacies). These vegetable oil scalp rubs should be used as frequently as needed to keep the scalp soft and comfortable without excessive oiliness; once or twice a week for most people.

Of course, vegetable oils taken internally are the best way to help lubricate your skin and scalp.

GIVE YOUR HAIR A CHANCE. Liquid foods send a stream of nourishment to your bloodstream which, in turn, feeds your scalp. You need much liquid food because it is estimated that you have an estimated 100,000 hairs constantly growing, shedding and replacing themselves on the scalp. When hair fails to replace itself, the root (or follicle) may be "thirsty" for the nutrients in live food juices. When a hair shaft (the visible extension of the root) is injured, step up your live food juice program to help the deficiency and to help the shaft become renourished to promote hair growth.

HAIR-RAISING HIGHLIGHTS OF CHAPTER 4:

1. Live food juices help correct hair distress.
2. Nature has four special steps to help improve metabolism and its related hair health.
3. The Hair-Growing Potion reportedly helped Leonard R.
4. Hair-Health Juice is easily made and has a powerhouse of scalp rejuvenation benefits.
5. Seed Juice and Seed Sprouts promote healthy young hair.
6. A unique ingredient in the Vitamin Hair-Growing Cocktail promotes hair bulb nutrition.
7. A Thirsty Thyroid is often in need of a special elixir that leads to improved hair health.
8. Use a natural bristle brush; eliminate white sugar and give your hair a fighting chance!

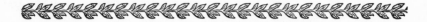

Chapter 5

How "Enzyme Cocktails" Can

Replenish Your Youthfulness

and Check Premature Aging

IF there is one special Youth Element created by Nature and nourished in plant foods it is the *enzyme*. Here is a dynamic source of health building power that promotes the look and feel of youth with almost no comparison in the world of Nature. In live food juices, enzymes can help check your aging factor and promote a vitalic zest for renewed living.

HOW ENZYMES HELP PROTECT AGAINST THE AGING PROCESS

Nature-Created Youth Builders. Enzymes are delicate youth-life building substances found in most living cells, especially in plant and seed foods. Each enzyme is an organized Nature-created substance which contains a vitamin, a mineral, and a specific protein. It may also be composed of a mineral, a hormone, and a specific protein. It may be a combination of vitamins, minerals, and hormones with a a specific protein. All ingredients within the minute-microscopic Nature-created enzyme work to help protect against the ravages of age.

Enzymes Promote Healing-Rejuvenation. Plant food enzymes are intimately connected with all healing and regenerative processes. Enzymes aid in your digestive functions, in turn, helping assimilation and elimination. They break down complex foods into simple substances which can be absorbed into your bloodstream to be sent to all body parts for nourishment and regeneration. Enzymes can quickly perform difficult internal biological processes, without energy or without themselves becoming involved in the change. For this reason, they are called *catalysts.*

The Youth Replenishment "Catalyst" Action of Enzymes. The seemingly self-regenerative power of enzymes which may seem like the secret of eternal life may well be in the *catalyst* action. That is, the enzyme performs an internal youthful replenishment action but does not become a part of the action itself. It does the work, then retreats and waits to do it again when needed. This may well be the legendary "Fountain of Youth" since Nature meant for enzymes to have eternal life.

How Enzymes Help Check the Aging Factor. Enzymes digest all food to make it small enough to pass through the minute pores of the intestine into the bloodstream. Enzymes help rebuild food into muscle, nerve, bone, or gland. Enzymes help in storing excess food in the liver or muscles for future use. Enzymes figure into the formation of urea to be eliminated in the urine, also in the elimination of carbon dioxide from the lungs. There is an enzyme to help build phosphorus into bone and nerve. Another enzyme helps fix iron into the red blood cells. Doctors have long known that in conditions of "tired blood" or anemic-like problems, it is insufficient to use iron-rich foods. Other factors are needed such as enzymes to metabolize the iron. Without the enzymes, all the iron in the world would not help correct the poor blood condition.

Enzymes Promote Natural Healing Processes. One enzyme

participates in the coagulation of the blood and thus stops bleeding. Another decomposes toxic hydrogen peroxide and liberates healthful oxygen for the body. One enzyme promotes oxidation (union of oxygen with other substances). Enzymes attack waste materials in the blood and tissues and transform them into urea and uric acid which may be easily eliminated.

Enzymes Nourish the Body and Mind. Enzymes change protein into assimilable amino acids; they transform fat or sugar into usable nourishing elements. Enzymes change carbohydrates into fat. Enzymes figure into all the vital processes of metabolism. Without enzymes, eaten food would lie in the system in a lump! With poor or weak enzyme supply, eaten food is inadequately metabolized and body decline may occur.

A Treasure of Enzymes Is Required for Youthful Health. There are close to a thousand known enzymes. Your body needs as many as possible because each enzyme acts upon *one* substance only. If you are weak, deficient or absent in *one* enzyme, it may well spell the difference between the look and feel of youth—or aging!

LOOK TO PLANT AND SEED JUICES FOR ENZYMES

In uncooked, raw, and non-processed plant and seed foods is the rich treasure of Nature-created enzymes. The juices squeezed from plants and seeds become a liberated treasure of these living substances. To obtain a goodly supply of enzymes, look to live food juices as Nature's own prepared sources.

Why Benjamin D. Could Not Correct Aging Defects with Juices. A construction engineer, Benjamin D. was frequently out in the field, on location sites, working long hours over blueprints and engineering schedules. A combination of overwork and improper eating left its toll on Benjamin. His face was crease-lined; his posture was stooped and he walked with the gait of an elderly man, even though he was in his very early 40's.

Benjamin D. was a victim of stomach pains, embarrassing constipation, and unsightly blemishes on his legs that threatened to become varicose veins. Similar blemished pigmentation appeared elsewhere on his body. Dust made him wheeze and sneeze. His eyes were bloodshot. He kept it a secret (even from his family) that his fingers were becoming stiff and he was threatened with arthritic distress. Benjamin D. was aging—rapidly.

The Wrong Source of Enzymes. Benjamin D. was unaware of the perishable factor of enzymes; namely, that processed foods destroy these miracle workers. He acquired many bottles and cans of mass-production and chemical-treated juices. None of them were of an organic source. He drank these juices regularly and while his thirst was satisfied, his health was not. He did not know that enzymes are killed in canning, pasteurizing, heating, cooking, baking, broiling, or frying. He did not know that many canned juices are first pre-heated and then pasteurized. These processes *kill* the enzymes so that while some nutrients are present, the precious life-substances are *not*. Benjamin D. developed bladder distress and soon had to submit to hospitalization. He could have had a new lease on prolonged health if he had consumed *live food juices* that are prime sources of youth-building enzymes.

THE "ENZYME COCKTAIL" THAT PUT YOUTH BACK INTO LIFE. Dorothy T. looked pleasant but she felt old. A few hours of ordinary housework would leave her exhausted and she would have to lie down and recuperate. Preparing the evening meal for her family was a chore that again required a rest period, even before she could tackle the dishes. Modern kitchen helps such as automatic washers and driers should have eased her burden, but they only made her more tired than before.

How Dorothy T. Corrected Her Enzyme Program. It came about that a local seed merchant in the farm community where she lived told her that she ought to feed her livestock (they lived on a farm) an abundance of raw seeds in the meal. The merrchant said the live seeds and uncooked or raw fruits and vegetables were rich in substances that would promote healthy and youthful livestock. If this was good for the livestock, Dorothy reasoned, it should be good for her, too. So she prepared this live food juice:

The "Young Again" Enzyme Cocktail

1 cup sunflower (hulled) or sesame seeds
1 cup cool water
(Blend well, first soaking.)
Add: 2 teaspoons honey
Sprinkle of sea salt
1/2 teaspoon of soya milk powder
2 cups water (or more, as thick or thin as desired)

Buzz in a blender until thoroughly assimilated. Drink one or more cups of this "Young Again" Enzyme Cocktail every single day. Dorothy T. liked to serve it over fresh *raw* fruits or stone-ground cereals, as well. This gave her a powerhouse of enzymes.

Benefits of Special "Young Again" Enzyme Cocktail: Dorothy T. found her strength returning slowly because the rich supply of Vitamin E in the seeds combined with the minerals in the honey and the amino acids in the protein. Together, the enzymes in these raw, uncooked foods joined to exert a metabolism that sent a supply of precious nourishment to the entire bloodstream. All vital body parts were bathed and nurtured with vital food elements that created a regeneration and a Look and Feel Of Youth that made Dorothy T. feel young again! Now, she drinks this cocktail twice daily, gives it to her family—and is as healthy as her livestock! Enzymes gave her a new lease on life. No longer does she require so many naps, no longer does she have cold fingers and toes and annoying sniffles when the weather changes. Now she is "young again." Thanks to enzymes.

POWER-PACKED ENZYME YOUTH TONIC

Here is a special all-natural tonic that is brimming with enzymes and other Nature-created nutrients that help revive and regenerate the system to promote the sought after Look and Feel of Youth:

6 tablespoons cold-pressed wheat germ oil
1/2 cup freshly squeezed carrot juice
1/2 cup freshly squeezed lettuce juice
1/4 cup freshly squeezed cucumber juice
2 tablespoons apple cider vinegar

Blend together as thoroughly as possible, using either a blender, a wire whisk or a spoon. Drink daily. It is suggested to drink this Power-Packed Enzyme Youth Tonic in the early afternoon when breakfast and lunch contents have been assimilated. Give the nutrients of this Youth Tonic a chance to work without interference.

Extra-Special Young Again Benefits of Power-Packed Enzyme Youth Tonic: The enzymes in the wheat germ oil join with those of the vegetables to promote these individual benefits to the body—they help promote an oxygen-sparing function. By maintaining the purity and availability of the oxygen in the system, the enzymes make it possible for every cell and fiber to function normally, to resist illness and to maintain youthful help.

Enzymes Resist Internal Aging. Internal aging is due to a process of oxidation. Since the enzymes and nutrients in this Youth Tonic work as a natural anti-oxidant, they help resist this process. The enzymes work to prevent the formation of free "radicals" (the medical name for debris that has accumulated and piled up in cellular membranes to cause aging disorders) and help serve as a built-in protection against accelerated aging. The enzymes and nutrients in the Youth Tonic promote this feeling of abundant health.

THE "SECOND CHANCE" OFFERED BY ENZYME POWER

Lester E. had undergone surgery. Physicians told him that he would be kept alive after the operation, and that he could expect a reasonable amount of life years thereafter. Lester E. hoped that he could have a "second chance" and live long enough to see his only daughter and only child in marriage. That was the most he could hope for.

Prospective Son-In-Law is Health Seeker. His prospective son-in-law was a natural health seeker. He was somewhat involved in taking yoga lessons, joining jogging clubs, physical fitness groups, and also in learning about natural foods. It was all part of his personalized program to put life into his years.

Suggests Enzymes. The young man suggested that his future father-in-law try corrective nutrition with emphasis on natural foods and enzymes. He said that since enzymes were the very core of life and health, they should form the foundation of the ailing man's struggle to live longer—and better—and younger. He insisted the ailing man eat large amounts of fresh raw fruits and vegetables. He also prepared the following:

Nu-Youth Enzyme Elixir

$1/4$ cup fresh orange juice
$1/4$ cup fresh grapefruit juice
$1/4$ cup fresh apple juice
2 tablespoons cold-pressed seed oil
2 tablespoons apple cider vinegar
Natural organic honey to taste

Mix vigorously with a blender, wire whisk or a spoon. Drink one glass about an hour *before* each of the three meals daily.

Unique Benefit of Nu-Youth Enzyme Elixir: The enzymes in these raw seed and plant foods work to create digestive power. The enzymes in the apple juice are especially beneficial in stimulating a flow of mouth enzymes so that foods could be better digested. The Magic Secret here is to drink the Nu-Youth Enzyme Elixir *before* eating a meal to prepare the digestive system, to perk it up into youthful enzymatic flow, and render digestion and assimilation a health-youth environment. Lester's problem was faulty digestion because of his surgery. Therefore, the program was to improve the digestive power with enzymes and help strengthen its ability to metabolize nutrients to promote the look and feel of youth. This special Elixir was a miracle in a glass—all Nature-created.

Lester E. Is Given a "Second Chance" by Enzyme Power. This corrective food program with emphasis on enzymes helped invigorate Lester so that his health enjoyed a comeback. He got his wish. He was healthy enough to see his only child get married. But once his daughter and her new husband were out of vicinity, Lester E. slid back to his previous faulty eating. He shrugged at the son-in-law's ideas; he discarded raw fruits and vegetables and the special Nu-Youth Enzyme Elixir. He began to decline in health. Like most people who feel a resurgence of vitality, he became flippant and self-assured and left the world of Nature. Lester did not live long enough to see the birth of his first grandchild. He had been given a second chance through Nature but had tossed it away.

SEVEN STEPS TO INCREASING YOUR ENZYME-YOUTH POWER

Many researchers have learned that a build-up of enzyme power adds up to prolonged youthful health. This is especially vital to those who reach the middle years. The reason here is that year after year of strain on the enzyme-secreting organs and glands have left them weak. It is especially true in folks who have eaten cooked or treated foods and who have denied themselves sufficient enzyme intake through raw foods. So to insure your intake of adequate and live enzymes, this simple rule of thumb is the foundation: eat raw foods that can be eaten raw; cook only those foods that must be cooked. Simple? Yet how many people shrug off such a simple program for increasing the enzyme-youth power?

This equally simple 7-step plan will help promote the supply of youth-maintaining enzymes in your body:

1. All fruits should be served raw, whenever possible. Frozen foods have temporarily inactivated enzymes so may be used in the absence of raw fruits. Canned fruits are enzyme-deficient.

2. All vegetables should be served raw, wherever possible. Use any seasonal vegetables in any desired salad form. Add a little raw cold-pressed wheat germ to further add to your enzyme supply. The only vegetables to be cooked are those which cannot be eaten raw Examples: potatoes, peas, squash, spinach, etc.

3. Begin a meal with a *raw* fruit or vegetable salad. This creates an internal "gushing of enzyme springs" to facilitate a youthful digestive power of assimilation.

4. Whenever possible, purchase, store and serve organically grown whole foods. Be sure to wash and cleanse all fruits and vegetables if they are purchased at a non-organic outlet.

5. Sprouting increases the enzymatic supply of seeds and grains. Sprouts should be served daily. Select organically grown seeds and grains from your nearest seed merchant.

6. Vitamins, minerals and enzymes are abundant in raw, certified milk and cream, raw buttermilk, and raw butter. Where these are permitted in the diet, use them in place of pasteurized or processed dairy products. If not permitted, then use *raw* nut milks or *raw* seed milks. You can make your own raw nut and seed milks by using a home mill machine (available at modest price at most health food stores). Run the nuts or seeds through the machine until they are like powder. Mix with water (spring water is suggested since it is free of contaminants and chemicals) and you have a power-packed enzyme beverage.

7. Enzymes are completely destroyed by heat if the food is subjected to a temperature beyond 120 F. degrees. Foods may be lightly cooked below this temperature when soaked and enjoy some enzyme preservation. Hence, the importance of *raw* foods.

THE "YOUTH SECRET" OF ENZYMES. If there is one beneficial "youth secret" of enzymes, it may well be this one—they help in the metabolization of the processes that control oxidation. This benefit helps ease the problem of cells turning "rancid." Enzymes then prevent the combining of oxygen with other substances that form the age-causing and somewhat fatal hydrogen peroxide "plaques" in the system that are known for speeding up cellular death. This may well be the "youth secret" of enzymes in their ability to check the aging factor.

YOUR ONE DAY ENZYME REJUVENATION PROGRAM

An office secretary, Jeanne T., finds it difficult to obtain fresh fruits and vegetables from the company cafeteria. Jeanne is troubled with a lack-lustre complexion as well as a feeling that might be summed up as loss of energy. She has one other problem that could be classified as *"claudication."* Namely, she feels a numbness in her legs and joints that is not painful—until she has to stand for a long time. She is unable to take medication because she develops a reaction. So Jeanne T. is able to derive partial self-rejuvenation and a reasonable restoration of supple limbs and joints by devoting one Saturday each week to this special Enzyme Rejuvenation Program:

BREAKFAST: Seasonal fresh raw citrus juice drink. This is freshly squeezed and non-processed to be certain it is rich in vitamins, minerals, and enzymes. Two glasses in the morning.

Breakfast Enzyme Booster Beverage: One hour after the above, Jeanne T. drinks a glass of seed or nut milk made with any available soya or nut powder mixed with bottled spring water. The benefit here is that this beverage exerts a "booster" to the morning enzymes because of the prime Vitamin E content that is known for entering the bloodstream and accelerating the circulation. Enzymes are promoted into this circulation to perform their miracle youth-corrective functions.

LUNCHEON: Two glasses of any seasonal fresh raw vegetable juices. If there are some hunger sensations, Jeanne T. then uses the pulp as part of a salad.

Luncheon Enzyme Renewal Punch: One hour after the above luncheon, Jeanne T. mixed together four tablespoons of wheat germ oil, two tablespoons of apple cider vinegar, and one cup of fresh tomato juice. The benefit here is that this combination contains valuable Vitamin E which acts as an energizer to the enzymes, and the potassium in the apple cider vinegar is used by enzymes to promote a self-cleansing action. Minerals in the tomato juice are assisted by the available enzymes to speed up circulation and nourish a sluggish bloodstream.

DINNER: Two glasses of any seasonal fresh raw vegetables. A cocktail of delicious live food juices. A sprinkle of wheat germ flakes. A teaspoon of lemon juice to produce a piquant flavour all its own. To ease any hunger urge, Jeanne T. will use the vegetable pulp for a salad.

Dinner Enzyme-Energizer Toddy. One hour after dinner, a cocktail of celery juice mixed together with two tablespoons of cold-pressed seed oil and a sprinkle of vegetized sea salt for flavour. The benefit here is that the celery juice revitalizes the still-sluggish enzymes that have not responded because it is a prime source of magnesium and iron. The cold-pressed seed oil is another prime source of enzymes; most important, it also has Vitamin E. This particular nutrient works together with Vitamin E in the celery juice and protects its store. Vitamin E in the seed oil also spares the health of Vitamin C in the juice. Both of these vitamins are sensitive to the presence of internal oxygen, but with Vitamin E in the digestive tract, sparing oxidation, the vitamins are preserved and able to perform youth-building functions. Hence the well-deserved name of Dinner Enzyme-Energizer Toddy.

JEANNE T. HELPS KEEP YOUNG ON THE ONE DAY ENZYME REJUVENATION PROGRAM. The special benefit of this "enzyme diet" program is that Jeanne T. does *not* eat anything else throughout the day so that these youth-building factors can perform their healing work without interference. Cooked foods in the digestive tract may ferment and inhibit the action of enzymes. Therefore, Jeanne T. has learned that it is a boost to her health to devote just one day a week to raw food juice intake. Her complexion improves and her leg aches are eased. She might enjoy more full rejuvenation if she could follow a natural raw-food program throughout the week but with company cafeterias being what they are, it is difficult. Others may be more fortunate and should take advantage of the availability of raw foods and enzymes.

ENZYMES OFFER HOPE FOR FREEDOM FROM PREMATURE AGING. Scientists are learning the magic power of enzymes. New weapons against aging include enzymes. Scientists know that one enzyme may help dissolve serious blood clots in the lungs. Another may be the sought-after key to the specific treatment and remission of certain forms of leukemia. Still another enzyme is believed to be the first specific anti-viral agent. Dentists have even begun using enzymes to correct tooth decay. Enzymes are known for being able to correct many errors in heredity and degenerative illnesses from mental retardation to senility.

Enzymes may well be regarded the physical embodiment of that *élan vital* or mystic force, by which some healers have attempted to define life.

Enzymes are needed to cause movement of muscles, the process of breathing, the storage of energy, the digestion and assimilation of food, the building of tissues, the course of reproduction, the transmission of nerve impulses, the workings of the brain *and even some of the thought processes themselves!*

ENZYMES: KEY TO YOUTHFUL LIFE. Enzymes are dynamic by offering a key to youthful life. Found almost totally in raw, non-processed live food juices made from fruits, vegetables, seeds and grains, enzymes should form the foundation in the program to reap the joys of the Look and Feel of Youth.

THE KEY TO UNLOCK THE MYSTERY OF PERPETUAL YOUTH. Enzymes may well be the key that will unlock the mystery and open the doorway to perpetual youth. Doctors have found enzyme imbalances and deficiencies in their study of aging. One of these problems is the decline of lactate dehydrogenase in skeletal muscles. Enzymes have been used to correct this age-causing illness. In the web of life's biochemical systems, enzymes are being used to help problems of hypertension, circulatory ailments, muscular distress, and convulsive disorders.

Where are these youth-building enzymes found? In the live food juices of living foods! Life builds life! Enzymes may well be the one Youth Element created by Nature and made available to you for the drinking!

IN REVIEW:

1. Enzymes are natural elements found exclusively in raw foods and their freshly squeezed juices. They serve to promote healing-rejuvenation and figure in nearly all life processes.

2. Enzyme cocktails help check the aging factor. Select fresh, raw juices rather than processed juices which was Benjamin D.'s error.

3. Dorothy T. felt a stream of rejuvenation with her "Young Again" Enzyme Cocktail. Takes minutes to make and offers an infinity of health.

4. The Power-Packed Enzyme Youth Tonic promotes internal youth.

5. Nu-Youth Enzyme Elixir prolonged Lester's health; it could have prolonged his life if he had continued the alliance with Nature.

6. Seven easy-to-follow steps help mobilize your enzyme-youth power.

7. A One Day Enzyme Rejuvenation Program created many benefits for Jeanne T.

8. Enzymes offer hope for freedom from aging and are considered the key to unlock the mysteries of perpetual youth. They're all-natural!

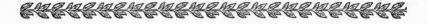

Chapter 6

How to Drink Your Vitamins to Cope

with Aging Arthritic Distress

To enjoy a long and youthful prime of life in your later years, you need supple, flexible, and resilient joints. Nature meant for you to have free-moving arms and legs, trouble-free back, energetic fingers and toes. Nature never meant for the human body to endure the prematurely aged problem of arthritis. Here is a distressful symptom of erroneous metabolism that requires immediate health attention. In Nature's arsenal of nutrients in liquid foods, there are many substances that have been seen to help correct the error in metabolism that brings on arthritic distress. By helping to correct the *cause* of arthritic distress, the symptoms become eased and there is a hopeful return to youthful flexibility. Nature has prepared reported relief in the form of live plant and seed juices.

HOW NOCTURNAL LEG CRAMPS WERE RELIEVED WITH SEED JUICE

Alfred T. was a victim of a familiar type of arthritic distress. He had nocturnal leg cramps that disturbed his slumber, caused an excruciating paroxysm of pain. In particular, he suffered severe arthritic-like pains in the calf of his leg. It was so painful that Alfred T. said he had to lie absolutely rigid, fearful of the slightest movement lest it further entangle the big traffic jam of nerves and muscles.

Seed Germ Oil Promotes Relief. When conventional medication did not give him the relief he sought, Alfred T. was told to try wheat germ oil. This all-natural seed juice is rich in *alpha tocopherol,* or Vitamin E, together with other vitamins that help promote its action in the system. Alfred T. began to take a special tonic: he would mix six tablespoons of wheat germ oil in a cup of freshly squeezed orange juice. He would drink one cup in the morning, one other cup at noontime, and a final cup at dinner time. He would drink these cups *before* the actual meal so that the nutrients could help promote their soothing action without interference of ingested foods.

Enjoys Relaxed and Youthful-Feeling Legs. After four weeks of this program, Alfred T. began to enjoy the feeling of relaxed legs. The Seed Germ Oil Tonic helped correct a mild deficiency or faulty metabolism that led to an insufficient blood circulation. Soon Alfred T. could enjoy a good night's sleep without any interference of arthritic-like pains. Nature, through the use of the Seed Germ Oil Tonic, helped ease his arthritic distress and promote a feeling of youthful legs.

"RESTLESS LEGS" RELAXED THROUGH FOOD JUICE. Mary E., at age 37, complained of having "restless legs" that plagued her for a period of ten years. The arthritic-like condition increased as it was neglected until Mary E. could not sleep. Now, with chronic insomnia, her general health began a decline. She felt certain she would soon become stricken with severe arthritis. She began looking for a drugless means of coping with her distress. Mary E. found that

Vitamin E in pure wheat germ oil could help promote a more wholesome circulation and also give her legs a feeling of ease and comfort. Mary E. took wheat germ oil, about five tablespoons daily, and also used it in salads. In conjunction with other natural health programs, she was able to obtain much desired relief. Her "restless legs" relaxed through the seed juice—wheat germ oil—and she was soon able to enjoy healthful sleep. Recovery was on the way.

WHY SEED JUICE IS BENEFICIAL TO ARTHRITIC DISTRESS. The combination of Vitamin E with other nutrients helps in improving the glycogen storage in the muscles. (Glycogen is a storage form of glucose that is formed by the liver.) It has been noted that in many arthritic patients there is a form of muscular constriction that is traced to improper glycogen storage. Vitamin E improves and regulates a healthful glycogen storage in the muscles; this, in turn, promotes a youthful resiliency to the limbs and helps relax and relieve the aging distress of arthritis. Wheat germ oil is just such a seed juice that helps promote this benefit.

ARTHRITIS: THIEF OF YOUTHFULNESS

Arthritis is regarded the oldest and most widespread chronic ailment and thief of youthfulness. The U.S. Public Health Service says some 13 million Americans are robbed of their young years by this ailment. About 600,000 are unable to work, perform household tasks, or carry on other activities because of arthritic distress.

Arthritis Wears Many Masks. Arthritis is a general encompassing term to describe over a hundred different disorders. As well as rheumatoid arthritis, they include gout, bursitis, lumbago, rheumatic fever, and osteoarthritis. The most common include rheumatoid arthritis and osteoarthritis. The latter is the bane of persons in their young 40's and causes a joint wearing-down that robs precious youthful years from life.

How to Help Correct Cause to Enjoy Relief. In addition to live food juices to help promote relief, it is essential to correct the cause. An arthritic attack may be an insidious health depletion traced to faulty metabolism over a long period of time, warranting attention. Or, an attack may be touched off by sprains, infections, joint injuries, emotional shocks, and even climate changes. Early symptoms that need correction include fatigue, pain, stiffness on arising, poor appetite, loss of weight, and a feverish condition. There may be recurring and periodic swelling of the joints. If neglected, arthritis may continue to cause the joints to be fused and engender possible permanent crippling. Prolonged neglect may cause the disease to affect the entire system, including the heart, lungs, blood vessels, kidneys, muscles, skin, and eyes.

Heed the Warning of Nature. Nature is wise to send warning symptoms that require immediate attention. These include persistent pain and stiffness on arising; pain, tenderness or swelling in one or more joints; recurrence of these symptoms; pain and stiffness in the lower back, knees and other joints; tingling sensations in fingertips; slight tingling in hands and feet; unexplained weight loss, fever, weakness or fatigue. Nature has sent these warnings that require swift correction to help bring about relief and less susceptibility to the ravages of age-causing arthritis.

HEALTH TONIC TO HEAL FIBROSITIS

Jenny R. was a victim of *fibrositis* (a form of arthritis in which there is inflammation of the white fibrous connective tissues that form muscle sheaths and merge into muscle attachments). When conventional medication only relieved the symptoms, she sought a natural health tonic. This consisted of a cold-pressed seed germ oil. She would mix a freshly squeezed glass of a vegetable juice with six tablespoons of wheat germ oil and drink it daily. In addition, Jenny R. corrected her other food intake and eliminated all bleached, devitalized foods. She also obtained sufficient nightly rest.

Jenny R. was soon able to enjoy so much more healing from this Seed Health Tonic that she discontinued it. Jenny R. felt a slight return of her arthritic-muscular distress, so she went back to the Seed Health Tonic and was able to have freedom from her age-causing problem. She continues with this daily dosage, and is able to enjoy the look and feel of youth— without arthritis distress. Nature helped her!

HOW LIVE FOOD JUICES HELP ESTABLISH HEALTHY MINERAL BALANCE

Andrew T. was troubled with a steadily increasing knife-like pain in his right shoulder blade. He noticed the pain kept on in its severity until he had to walk with a slight slump to help the pressure. He tried medication with some beneficial relief of pain. But when he discontinued the medication, his arthritic pain returned and it was much more severe than before! The medication had dulled the pain but the arthritis was allowed to increase in its insidious way. Now, Andrew T. felt pain in both shoulder blades.

Errs in His Food Juice Program. In an effort to help resist the ravages of this type of arthritis, Andrew T. eliminated unnatural foods, performed regular exercises and then started a program of fruit and vegetable juices. But he did not experience the coveted relief. In fact, he felt worse than before!

His mistake: he obtained mass production supermarket bottled and canned juices that were saturated with additives, preservatives, sugars, and sweeteners. It was this excessive consumption of sugar that caused an error in his metabolism that increased his arthritis distress.

Andrew T. did not believe that bleached sugar could be responsible for his problem and he gave up. In a while, he was doubled over with seemingly irreversible arthritic distress. This could have been averted if he had selected natural live food juices that were freshly squeezed; or, he should have selected bottled and canned juices at a health store, where labels should read "No Sugar Added." It could have made a lot of difference!

Mineral Balancing Power in Live Food Juices. Minerals and vitamins in live food juices work to help stabilize the all-important calcium-phosphorus ratio in the blood. Any alteration can lead to arthritic distress, among other problems. Sugar-free live food juices help promote a natural balance of calcium-phosphorus and establish a healthful and youthful body chemistry.

Sugar-Free Program Soothes Arthritic Distress. Refined foods and commercially prepared juices are usually saturated with white sugar. This consumption of white sugar displaces the body chemistry balance, and further upsets the delicate calcium-phosphorus balance. Refined sugar boosts calcium but it lowers phosphorus. When this effect has worn off, the reverse occurs, with the phosphorus shooting up and the calcium becoming depressed. Accordingly, the effect is felt in mental depression that accompanies arthritic and limb stiffening known as a form of rheumatism. Hence drinking juices that are saturated in refined sugar can have a serious effect. The problem with Andrew T. is that he did not select natural juices. His mineral balance was so distorted that his symptoms increased. White sugar was the villain.

RAW JUICE PROGRAM RESTORES FREEDOM OF FLEXIBLE JOINTS. A reported case is that of Norma C. At age 52, she fell victim to arthritis. Upon examination, it was found that she had a serious mineral imbalance. She ate refined foods, drank six cups of coffee daily with much sugar in each, two cocktails and a highball. Furthermore, Norma C. abused her system by eating candy, cookies, and canned fruits. All of these "foods" had much white sugar. Her arthritis increased until she was doubled over with pain.

Norma C. was taken off the white sugar regimen. All foods containing white sugar were eliminated. She was given a Raw Juice Program in which freshly squeezed fruit juices and vegetable juices were taken daily. She followed this special Raw Juice Program for three months. Then, when her calcium-phosphorus level was stabilized, her arthritis pains melted and she felt flexible joints again. She was young—at 52. Raw juices had put life into her limbs!

FRUIT JUICES PROVIDE "FOOD" FOR
THE CARTILAGE

Many physicians have found that live fruit juices are sources of "food" for the cartilage. The benefit here is in Vitamin C that is found in fresh and non-processed live fruit juices.

Good Sources: Oranges, lemons, grapefruits, tangerines, grapes, plums, currants, apricots, cherries, berries.

How Vitamin C Promotes Joint Youth: Vitamin C assists in the formation of collagen for the maintenance of integrity and stability of the connective tissues, and this includes the bones, cartilage, muscles, and vascular tissues. Collagen is helped by the Vitamin C in fresh fruit juices. Collagen is the substance that is so important in all connective tissue—it is the material that makes gelatin when you boil bones. A deficiency of Vitamin C leads to instability and fragility of all such tissue; it leads to a breakdown of intercellular cement substance, resulting in easy rupture of any and all of these connective tissues; this includes the discs of the backbone, the ligaments and small sacs in the interior of the joints *and the cartilage which helps in the movement of joints.* The vulnerability of these joints may be, then, the underlying cause for arthritic distress.

Your Vitamin C Health Cocktail

$^1/_2$ cup grapefruit juice
$^1/_4$ cup orange juice
$^1/_4$ cup apricot juice
2 tablespoons rose hips powder
(sold at health food stores).

Mix vigorously and drink an hour before breakfast; mix a fresh Vitamin C Health Cocktail again and drink an hour before lunch. Your third Vitamin C Health Cocktail is taken an hour before dinner. This helps boost your much-needed Vitamin C supply to feed your cartilage and help relieve the problems of arthritis.

BIOFLAVONOID TONIC FOR ARTHRITIC DISORDERS

The bioflavonoids are little-known but highly beneficial food substances that are found in fruits, along with Vitamin C. It is this *combination* in a live food juice that is known for helping promote a youthful flexibility of joints.

Plant Food Sources: A Nature-created *combination* of bioflavonoids and Vitamin C will be found in lemons, grapes, plums, black currants, grapefruit, apricots, cherries, and blackberries.

Most Potent Source: The golden orange contains some 1000 milligrams of bioflavonoids as well as a powerhouse of Vitamin C.

Plant Juice is Powerful: The bioflavonoids are found in concentrated form in the white skin and segment part of the orange and the selected fruit. Hence, juicing will release this treasure of nutrient supply so that it can enter into the composition of your capillaries and the cellular walls of the limbs.

Nature's Bioflavonoid Tonic

1/2 cup freshly squeezed orange juice
1/2 cup freshly squeezed grape juice
1 teaspoon lemon juice
2 tablespoons dark organic honey

Stir vigorously and drink promptly.

Benefits of Bioflavonoid Tonic: Approximately 1000 milligrams of bioflavonoids in the tonic help nourish the capillaries and blood vessels of the body. They further promote a flexibility of the arterial walls and scour the accumulated joints to help create a youthful suppleness of limbs. It would be wise to drink the tonic three or more times daily, to ingest at least 3000 milligrams of the bioflavonoids that are needed by the body.

JENNY R. FINDS NEW HOPE FOR ARTHRITIS RELIEF THROUGH BIOFLAVONOIDS. At age 52, Jenny R. suffered from rheumatoid arthritis in both hands, wrists and elbows and in the right shoulder, knees and ankles. It is reported that treatment consisted of being given 3000 milligrams of bioflavonoids. In 7 days, she "felt better." In two weeks, the pain had practically gone. She showed improved digestion and normal bowel action. Her blood pressure dropped from 190 to 176. Five weeks of Bioflavonoid Tonics and Jenny R. now had more action in her joints and more endurance than she had known in several years. This was a very severe case with crippling changes in the joints. The Bioflavonoid Tonic treatment brought about improvement that doctors described as "dramatic." Live food juices had helped her cope with the vanishing arthritis.

LEG ARTHRITIS RELIEVED WITH BIOFLAVONOIDS. Much is said about bursitis, which is also known to be a form of arthritis. Live food juices with bioflavonoids helped one 38 year-old man. John T. suffered from severe sub-patellar (knee-joint) bursitis. He had extensive local swelling, local heat, extreme tenderness, severe pain and limitation of motion. John T. began to take a live food juice that gave him a total of 600 milligrams a day of bioflavonoids. (The juice of one fresh orange should supply this amount.) It is reported that the swelling and pain were almost completely gone in 24 hours with this live food juice program. In 72 hours, the lesion had subsided, leaving only slight local tenderness. The bioflavonoids relieved and corrected his arthritis distress and he could walk again—free from bursitis pain!

SEED JUICE HELPS REDUCE DRUG REQUIREMENT

A high supply of Vitamin E (available from sunflower seed oil) helped improve a woman's arthritis so that she was subsequently able to reduce her drug requirement.

At age 29, Mrs. R. T. suffered from arthritis of the elbows, arms, fingers and legs. She was given high steroid doses which eased the symptoms but did not correct the cause. Doctors hoped she was recovering from arthritis so reduced Mrs. R.

T.'s amount of steroid drugs. The arthritis symptoms returned with such severity that she could scarcely walk.

Seed Juice Promotes Recovery. The doctors then gave Vitamin E (the same potency as found in four tablespoons of sunflower seed oil) together with a reduced steroid. Now, the housewife, Mrs. R. T., could be active enough to the point of folk dancing and bicycle riding. When last heard of, the steroid dose was further reduced and the seed juice increased and Mrs. R. T. was able to have flexible limbs again. Perhaps she may soon give up her drugs and turn to the seed juice for correction of her arthritis.

Benefit of Seed Juice: The Vitamin E and the unsaturated fatty acids in sunflower seed oil have the ability to duplicate the benefits of drugs in easing symptoms. Vitamin E then is able to stimulate the blood circulation in the fingers and toes. It is reported by some doctors that many of their arthritic patients no longer had a "cold feeling" in their limbs when seed juices supplemented steroids.

Here we see that a combination of natural ingredients in live food juices from plants and seeds helps bring about corrective healing of metabolic disorders.

Arthritis is often believed to be brought about by an impaired mechanism that upsets the normal balance inside the body cell. It begins with a deficiency of oxygen in the cell and then goes on to destroy the cell.

Juices Control Cellular Oxygen. Live food juices from plants and seeds control the oxygen content of cells. By using these juices, you help give your cells the oxygen required. Furthermore, live plant and seed juices help promote collagen. This is an albuminoid—a *protein* made of amino acids. So we can well understand the value of a balanced program of *all* live food juices that work in harmony to manufacture the collagen that is found in the bone, cartilage, tendons, and skin. Many rheumatic disorders have been traced to degenerative changes in the collagen. A live food juice will send a stream of essential Vitamin C, bioflavonoids, amino acids, and Vitamin E to the joints so that bundles of healing collagen may be speedily formed.

THREE BENEFITS OF FOOD JUICES FOR ARTHRITIC RELIEF

There are three special benefits made possible through live food juices that are of special value to the arthritic:

1. Helps increase elimination of waste products through the skin and kidneys by improved metabolism.

2. Improved circulation of the blood and other body fluids because nutrients in the live plant and seed juices promote healthy blood vessels.

3. Gentle dissolution of adhesions and the softening of any thickening in muscles and tissues.

Added up: nutrients help relieve joint stiffness, loosening sore muscles and helping to promote a freer motion.

It is essential to build a live food juice program into your search for the Look and Feel of Youth as early as possible. Arthritic-stricken muscles are forced to be inactive and this causes them to become less and less usable. This leads to less and less activity and, consequently, more and more pain with decreased mobility. The longer you delay, the more difficult is the road to recovery. Look to Nature for youthful joints and a youthful health!

BASIC POINTS IN REVIEW:

1. Nocturnal leg cramps were reportedly eased with a simple seed juice. Alfred T. felt "young legs" again.

2. Special oil helps Mary E. relax her "restless legs."

3. Seed Health Tonic promotes relief for Jenny R.'s fibrositis.

4. Sugar additives in Andrew's juices created serious consequences.

5. Arthritis relief is possible with special mineral balance power available through fresh live juices.

6. A Vitamin C Health Cocktail is food for the cartilage.

7. Little-known Bioflavonoid Tonic promotes amazing benefit.

8. Seed juices reduce need for drugs.

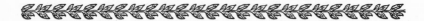

Chapter 7

How to Feel Like a "Young Blood"

Again with Natural Mineral Tonics

CHARLES T. was embarrassed to shake hands. His
fingers were cold and clammy and sent a shiver to the
recipient of his handclasp. Furthermore, when he embraced
his children, he made them squirm and grimace because his
hands were so uncomfortably cold. His condition was accom-
panied by increasing chilliness and a tingling sensation in his
fingertips and toes, as well. Charles T. not only felt "old" at
44, but he looked "old" with a waxen complexion, pale lips,
and crease-lined face. He was diagnosed as having a poor
blood circulation. Medication caused a reaction and he could
not take drugs. His "tired blood" distress made him feel cold
in weather when everyone went in their shirtsleeves. Not
Charles. He had to wear a sweater!

NATURAL MINERAL TONIC PROMOTES BLOOD CIRCULA-
TION. Charles T. endured his condition with stoic silence. He
might have continued on in his health decline which could

have led to assorted related disorders, had not the family decided to do some housecleaning. He came across some notes written by his grandmother, describing some old-fashioned spring tonics she would give to the children to help improve their blood health. There was one that his grandmother said would "whip up the blood and make you feel like a Young Blood at any age." It interested Charles and he made the following tonic:

"YOUNG BLOOD" MINERAL TONIC. Mix one-half cup of freshly squeezed grape juice with one-half cup of raisin juice. Add one teaspoon of lemon juice. Mix in one teaspoon of apple cider vinegar. Stir vigorously. Drink one tall glass an hour before *each* of the three daily meals. The benefit is to permit the power-packed iron and potassium content of these food juices to work upon the circulation without interference. Three glasses daily for a week would help stir up circulation through mineralization of the bloodstream.

Charles T. Gets Color in His Face and Warmth in His Fingers. It took two full weeks before Charles T. felt warmth in his fingers and toes. His skin color improved. A bloom appeared on his cheeks. Crease lines melted away. Now he could shake hands with warm confidence and play with his children without being embarrassed about how "cold" he felt. He continues with this "Young Blood" Mineral Tonic and feels as young as he looks—thanks to Nature and grandmother!

HOW MINERALS IN LIVE FOOD JUICES PROMOTE HEALTHIER BLOOD

Minerals in live food juices work upon the system to promote a healthier bloodstream that, in turn, creates a look and feel of youth. Here are five basic benefits of minerals in these live food juices:

1. *Promotes Youthful Oxygenation.* Minerals in the bloodstream help promote the absorption of oxygen in the lungs, distributing it to every organ and every part of the body; the

mineral-enriched bloodstream then takes on a cargo of carbon dioxide wastes which it returns to the lungs for disposal.

2. *Self-Cleansing Benefit.* Minerals regulate the process of self-cleansing. They cause the bloodstream to carry other waste products from the body tissues to the kidneys, which filter out the wastes into the urine.

3. *Creates Internal Nourishment for Look and Feel of Youth.* Minerals send the blood streaming through the body channels; they enable the blood to gather up nutrients and water from the digested food in the intestines and to feed these nutrients to the tissues and cells, nourishing them and helping to promote the look and feel of youth.

4. *Regulate Vital Hormone Balance.* Minerals transport hormones or "chemical messengers" from the body glands to other parts where they serve to keep you looking young through adequate glandular balance.

5. *Maintain Healthful Temperature.* Minerals enter into the bloodstream to help regulate body temperature, promoting a feeling of youthful warmth to fingers and toes and other extremities. Many so-called "chills" may be due to poor mineral supply. Look to natural live food juices for mineral tonics to regulate a healthful body temperature.

YOUTH-BUILDING POWER OF MINERAL TONICS. Mineral tonics are not only highly important to the well-being of the entire body, but they are of especial importance to the local structures of the bowel—the glands lining it, the muscles forming its walls and the nerves controlling and directing these structures. Mineral tonics help protein to form, enable the vagus nerve that controls stomach activity to function, influence muscle contraction and nerve response, and control body liquids to permit youthful nourishment to pass into the bloodstream.

Mineral Tonics Promote Healthful Digestion. Mineral tonics help in digestion and are required for your physiological processes. Skeletal rigidity and strength require minerals; the oxygen-carrying function of the blood is sparked by mineral tonics. There may also be a condition of intestinal stasis—that is, a reduction of the peristaltic contractions of the stomach, needed for proper digestion, if you are mineral-deficient. A healthy digestion promotes a look and feel of youth. Mineral tonics offer you this opportunity.

Caution: Deficiency Is Unwise. In the absence of minerals, the bacteria of putrefaction multiply with enormous rapidity in the slowed-down current of food waste matter passing down the canal of the bowel. They not only produce poisons that pass into the blood and burden the organ of elimination, but they locally irritate and ultimately set up an inflammatory state in the lining of the bowel, called colitis. This is the start of internal aging. A deficiency is unwise.

MINERAL TONICS WITH LIVE FOOD JUICES

To promote internal youthfulness through mineral tonics, here are old-time, all-natural live food juices you can prepare in your own home, for a modest cost, in a brief time to promote a feeling of being a "young blood":

STRONG BONE MINERAL TONIC. Susan U. developed problems of brittle bones. As a librarian, she found it difficult to carry small amounts of books. If she bumped against a shelf, she had aches for days. She was obviously deficient in calcium, the mineral in the blood that is needed to be stored inside the ends of the bones in long, needle-like crystals called *trabeculae.* Here is Susan U.'s Strong Bone Mineral Tonic:

Mix one-half cup of soy bean milk together with freshly squeezed lettuce juice. Add one-half cup of celery juice. Stir vigorously. Drink daily.

Susan's benefit: The rich supply of natural calcium and phosphorus in this Strong Bone Mineral Content worked together to help feed the skeletal structure, promote a healthful storage depot and, in turn, promote strong, youthful bones. It took several months of regular tonic drinking before she no longer bruised so easily and was able to enjoy stronger bone health.

MINERAL ENERGY TONIC. Co-workers scoffed at Julius E. who would take a "coffee break" with his all-natural Mineral

Energy Tonic. This bookkeeper for a large factory was anxious to boost his energy supply. He noted that coffee would give a boost but was quickly followed by a mid-afternoon letdown. So he relied upon three special mineral-rich vegetables that provided a powerhouse of energy through high phosphorus content. He prepared equal portions of freshly squeezed carrot, celery, and radish juices. He added two tablespoons of onion juice because of the enzyme that helped the other three juices become speedily assimilated. This formed Julius' Mineral Energy Tonic. He used one cup during his "coffee break" and returned to work with youthful vitality. His co-workers fell into a slump. Julius could even work overtime and this gave him a coveted promotion. His co-workers were jealously left behind. They laughed at Nature and reaped the consequences.

The benefit here is that the rich phosphorus in the three vegetables (carrot, celery, and radish) worked in the form of juice to convert oxidative energy into cellular work. The minerals in this special Mineral Energy Tonic then helped in contraction of muscles, secretions of glands, functions of internal organs, and, most essential, in generation of nerve impulses. The unique benefit of the Mineral Energy Tonic is in its power to metabolize fats and starches and promote a youthful energy fuel. All of this through live food juices.

BLOOD ENRICHMENT MINERAL TONIC. Mix together one-half cup of raisin juice, one-half cup of apricot juice, and a spoonful of lemon juice. Drink several cups daily. Here is a power-packed mineral tonic that is a prime source of iron. This live food juice puts iron and oxygen into your body tissues and muscle cells. The special benefit of this Blood Enrichment Mineral Tonic is in its supply of iron which enters into the hemoglobin, the oxygen-carrying pigment of the red blood cells. This helps nourish the bloodstream, warming the extremities and giving a healthful skin color. There are over 5 million red cells in just one cubic millimeter of blood, and iron is required for each and every cell. Feed the cells the needed iron with this live food juice made right in your own home.

MIND-BOOSTING MINERAL TONIC. Sluggish mentality may have labelled Ralph R. as a "mental defective." Although he was in his early teen years, he was doing so poorly in schoolwork that he was in a class for youngsters not even ten years of age! Ralph R. was tested and examined and while nothing organic was found to be the cause, a blood test showed that he was extremely deficient in iodine. An alert nutritionist suggested this special iodine tonic that would help improve his glandular function and thereby revive his mental abilities: Mix together equal portions of freshly squeezed red cabbage juice with tomato juice. Drink as often as possible. For added impact, stir in one-half teaspoon of sea salt or kelp (available at most health food stores) which sends a stream of ocean-rich minerals into the bloodstream.

The special benefit of this Mind-Boosting Mineral Tonic is that it feeds the thyroid gland through its iodine content. This mineral enables the thyroid to manufacture thyroxin, the hormone that stimulates emotional vigor. In young Ralph's situation, the molecule of iodine was speedily snatched from the bloodstream by the thyroid gland to manufacture this all-essential hormone, thyroxin.

It took a month of special iodine-intake to help improve his emotional stability. He soon recovered and was able to advance in his schoolwork and catch up with the other youngsters. He now drinks three Mind-Boosting Mineral Tonics daily to give his bloodstream the youthful transportation power it requires to nourish his glands.

THE POWER OF A POTASSIUM COCKTAIL

One live food juice may well stand out above others for its "young blood" power of minerals. This particular live food juice is a miracle source of *potassium*—the single mineral that helps to promote the look and feel of youth throughout your bloodstream.

HOW TO MAKE YOUR POTASSIUM COCKTAIL. Select sun-dried fruits such as apricots, prunes, raisins, pears, and peaches. Be sure to obtain sun-dried fruits that have *not* been chemically dried or treated. These are available at health stores.

Heat a kettle of water. After it bubbles, turn off heat and let the water simmer down. Next, place an assortment of sun-dried fruits in a deep bowl. Cover with the simmered water. Place a cover on the bowl. *Let remain at room temperature overnight.* In the morning, pour off one or two cups of the juice and drink. This is your Potassium Cocktail. You may eat the fruit for breakfast. This Potassium Cocktail has a power-packed mineral benefit that is reportedly second to none for its effectiveness in rejuvenating the bloodstream and re-creating the sought-after look and feel of youth. Here are the *six* basic benefits of the Potassium Cocktail:

1. *Establishes Regularity.* The minerals in the Potassium Cocktail promote a smooth bulk which has an emollient effect in the intestine. They also contain a *natural* laxative principle. This principle is heat-stable and water soluble, hence is carried over into the Potassium Cocktail.

2. *Enriched Vitamin Supply.* This mineral tonic is a valuable source of Vitamin A and also has beneficial amounts of thiamine, riboflavin, niacin, and the B-complex nutrients. All work in harmony to promote vitamin nourishment of the bloodstream.

3. *Promotes Youthful Energy.* The unique blending of minerals with strong potassium supply helps promote youthful energy. The Potassium Cocktail is rich in the quickly assimilable fruit sugars, dextrose, and levulose.

4. *Stabilizes Blood Levels.* The mineral tonic has Nature-created ingredients in a healthful balance. There are good amounts of calcium, phosphorus, and iron, and a low sodium content. This helps stabilize a youthful blood level.

5. *Restores Youthful Blood.* The Potassium Cocktail promotes hemoglobin potency and red cell restoration, the key to youthful blood. Nutrients work to invigorate the iron and copper balance, as well.

6. *Maintains Youthful Alkaline Reserve.* The Potassium Cocktail helps maintain a normal oxygen-combining power of

blood plasma; it also maintains the hydrogen ion concentration of the urine in normal health. All this is possible through healthful potassium which works with other vitamins and enzymes to promote youthful invigoration. The Potassium Cocktail's unique blood-building benefit is in its regulation of the acid-alkaline reserve that is the root of the program to look and feel young again.

DRINK YOUR WAY TO NEW YOUTH. A Potassium Cocktail helps you drink your way to a new youthful feeling. Potassium helps activate your kidneys in disposing of body waste substances and controls body fluids and essential physiological and metabolic processes. This all-natural folk remedy is a Mineral Tonic that helps you enjoy life—at any age.

BEAUTY MINERAL TONIC

Gladys E. had a sluggish bloodstream. It showed in her unsightly blue streaked, raised veins, "goose bumps on her flesh," and strained features. Gladys E. looked waxen in appearance. The problem was worsened by the fact that Gladys E. was a beautician at a leading salon that was supposed to offer beauty and glamour through makeup. How could Gladys E. arouse confidence in clients when she looked haggard and worn?

Client's Husband Shows Her the Way to Mineral Beauty. She was giving a facial to a healthy looking woman who had brought her husband along with her. Gladys E. noted the youthful appearance of the woman (and her husband, too) and knew that both were much older than she. She started talking about it and learned, from the husband, that the secret was in fresh juices that had a rich supply of sulphur. Here was a mineral that had the power to so invigorate the bloodstream that age-causing bacteria could be resisted. The client's husband suggested the following:

BEAUTY MINERAL TONIC: Mix equal portions of cranberry juice, pineapple juice, and seasonal berry juice. Add a sprinkle of lemon juice. Mix vigorously and drink at a time when the digestive system is free from the presence of other foods. This helps the sulphur promote bile secretions and enables the liver to absorb other minerals that would spur the protein metabolism and body oxidative processes. This unusual combination of benefits made this mineral tonic a sought-after source of youth promotion. This Beauty Mineral Tonic provided nourishment, via the bloodstream, to the skin, nails, and cellular tissues as well. Several glasses daily would help promote a sulphur foundation in the system.

Gladys E. Looks Better in Three Weeks. It took three weeks of the Beauty Mineral Tonic (two glasses daily) to help promote mineral enrichment of the bloodstream. Soon she had a youthful pinkish glow, roses in her cheeks, and better health. However, she did not regulate the time when the Mineral Beauty Tonic was to be taken. She erred in deciding that it made no difference when she had the tonic. It would work anyway. She consumed it on a full stomach and her over-worked liver had to put aside the minerals and create faulty assimilation. Two months later, she looked worse than before. She gave up. She felt that the minerals were just false hopes. She could have enjoyed the look and feel of youth through this Mineral Tonic if she had cooperated. All Gladys E. had to do was drink it on an empty stomach so that the sulphur could promote health without interference. But, she resisted. She lost!

HOW MINERAL TONICS INVIGORATE BLOOD CELLS AND RELIEVE ANEMIA

Anemia is a common disorder. The average anemic person looks pale. This is a condition in which there are too few red cells in the blood, or too little hemoglobin in the cells, or both. The anemic person usually has only vague symptoms of ill health. Often, he is thought to be "plain lazy" or a "chronic complainer."

Prolonged Mineral Deficiency May Deplete Health. A prolonged mineral deficiency reduces the numbers of red blood cells. Also, there is a deficiency of hemoglobin in the cells and the body breakdown begins. There is more than just poor skin color. There is the inability to enjoy natural healing of common problems; wounds do not properly heal and infectious allergic conditions appear to linger on. The cold feeling is pronounced. Headaches and depression are common disorders. This is Nature's signal to increase mineral content.

THE ALL-NATURAL IRON TONIC. Mix together three tablespoons *unflavored* gelatin powder and two tablespoons of desiccated liver powder in one cup of tomato juice. Use a sprinkle of lemon juice for added flavor. Drink three glasses daily, preferably an hour before mealtime.

Benefits: The gelatin powder is a powerhouse of amino acids; these work upon the dynamic iron source of the desiccated liver and join with the minerals in the tomato juice to help perform a synergistic action upon the bloodstream. The minerals in this All-Natural Iron Tonic enter into the hemoglobin and also become stored in the spleen and liver. The minerals further nourish the bloodstream to create *fibrin,* a substance that helps clot wounds and promote better healing. Without fibrin, a person could bleed to death from a single scratch! Minerals create this lifesaver.

Drink All-Natural Iron Tonic Regularly. The earlier you provide minerals to your bloodstream, the more effective will be the benefits. Many of us cling to the delusion that an "anemic condition" is the same thing as an indoor pallor which will clear up in the sunshine. True, sunshine helps stimulate circulatory flow, but it is only *part* of your health quest. Poor blood problems can occur in the summer as well as the winter. Use mineral tonics to help build up a healthy bloodstream. An All-Natural Iron Tonic is vital to promote the look and feel of youth.

NATURE'S SOURCE OF ABUNDANT MINERAL TONICS. Basically, Nature has put blood-building minerals in fresh citrus fruits and also raw vegetables. Good supplies of most minerals will be found in oranges, grapefruits, red and black berries, raisins, prunes, apricots (a highly potent source), plums, and peaches. Vegetables include turnips, radishes, kale, artichokes, red cabbage, lettuce, tomato, beet tops, watercress, and cucumbers.

Blackstrap Molasses an Old-Time Mineral Source. Granny was wise in giving the youngsters a special Granny Mineral Tonic in early spring. She mixed blackstrap molasses together with any seasonal fruit juice and gave them to the youngsters. The reasoning here is that during the long confinement of winter, the mineral supply may have weakened. Spring called for physiological adaptation and a greater mineral nourishment to meet that need. Granny was wise. The youngsters—and Granny—had the look and feel of youth with the molasses and fruit juice combination.

WHY A SEED JUICE IS A VALUABLE BLOOD FOOD. Marilyn T. has always used wheat germ oil to enrich her bloodstream. She has a young look; she has roses in her cheeks. Her skin is warm and soft as a peach. Marilyn T. is 58. At one time she had developed unsightly skin blotches, caught one cold after another, was bent over and walked with a stooped gait. Then she was told that seed juice—or natural seed oils—could promote a feeling of rejuvenation. She changed her diet to include natural foods, and made it a rule of thumb to use this simple Seed Juice Tonic every single day:

Seed Juice Tonic for Healthy Blood: Mix four tablespoons of wheat germ oil (or any seed oil) together with a cup of tomato juice. Sprinkle with sea salt, if desired. Drink daily.

Benefit: The Vitamin E in the wheat germ oil combines with minerals and works to prevent too-rapid oxidation (burning or metabolism) of nutrients and helps keep unsaturated fatty acids from producing age plaques (toxic peroxides and hydrocarbons) in the metabolic process. The Seed Juice Tonic helps keep the blood pure and young. It works to promote the process of *hematopoiesis*—the synthesis of young red blood cells. It works to rejuvenate the bloodstream. It helped Marilyn T. correct her lifetime of ill blood health and now she looks a younger-than-young 58.

MIX YOUR OWN MINERAL TONICS. Select any seasonal fruits and combine them to prepare an old-fashioned but highly successful Mineral Tonic. Also, select seasonal vegetables and mix a Blood Building Cocktail that will promote youthful cellular oxidation and ease the formation of age plaques. In Marilyn T.'s situation, many of the blotches faded as her skin color returned through an enriched mineral-fed bloodstream. The Seed Juice Tonic promoted this healing process.

FEED YOUR BLOODSTREAM A LOOK-AND-FEEL-YOUNG-AGAIN MINERAL TONIC. When minerals enter the bloodstream, they help promote vital body functions. They send nutrients via the bloodstream to all body parts. They maintain an acid-alkaline balance, regulate hormonal flow, stabilize your nervous system, neutralize wastes, help in elimination, wash and regenerate millions of blood cells. To feel like a "Young Blood" look to Mineral Tonics.

IN REVIEW:

1. "Young Blood" Mineral Tonic put color in Charles' face and gave him warm hands and feet and a "young again" feeling.

2. Mineral Tonics help promote five basic benefits.

3. A Strong Bone Mineral Tonic helps nourish the skeletal structure.

4. A special Mineral Energy Tonic gave Julius E. the stamina to work overtime when others faded into ill health.

5. Simple Blood-Enrichment Mineral Tonic eases problems of anemic disorders.

6. Ralph R. was relieved of "mental defective" problems with a Mind-Boosting Mineral Tonic.

7. A Potassium Cocktail offers six power-packed blood health benefits.

8. A Beauty Mineral Tonic may give you roses in your cheeks—by Nature and not cosmetics.

9. Granny's Mineral Tonic is effective when used daily.

10. Seed Juice is a little-known but valuable blood food that puts a "dynamite action" into minerals you eat.

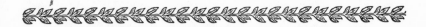

Chapter 8

How to Drink Your Proteins and Nourish

Your "Younger-Feeling" Amino Acids

TAKE a look at yourself in the mirror! What do you see? A magnificent package of protein. All that shows—your skin, hair, nails, and eyes—is made of protein. Your teeth, too, contain amounts of protein.

Much of what you do *not* see is also protein—your blood and lymph, your heart and lungs, tendons and ligaments, brain and nerves and just about the rest of you is made of protein. Genes, those strange regulators of heredity, are a form of protein. Hormones, the mysterious controllers of bodily functions and processes, and enzymes, the sparkplugs of metabolism, also are protein.

Next to water, protein is the most plentiful substance in the body. If all the water were squeezed out of you, most of your dry weight would be protein. About a third of the protein is in the muscle. About a fifth is in the skin. The rest is in the other tissues and body fluids. There are several dozen proteins in the bloodstream alone.

One of the busiest blood proteins is hemoglobin, which constantly transports oxygen from the lungs to the tissues and brings carbon dioxide back from the tissues to the lungs. Ninety-five per cent of the hemoglobin molecule is protein. The other five per cent is the portion that contains the iron. Protein is Nature's life fluid to help promote the look and feel of youth. In the form of seed and plant juices, protein has several distinct advantages:

1. *Speedily Assimilated.* The released protein is made readily available for the system to speedily assimilate.

2. *Increased Value to Health.* Liquid juices that are rich in protein have an increased value to the body. The protein has been liberated from tough, fibrous woody pulps, stems, leaves, and stalks, and has a powerhouse of nourishment to the body.

3. *More Amino Acids Available in Juice.* The metabolism of the body may be weak and unable to extract amino acids during the digestive process. Therefore, live food juices have available amino acids to help spare extra digestive effort. Otherwise the food pulp might remain incompletely digested and pass off with the un-released amino acids still intact. Live food juices release these amino acids and make them easily available for your Look and Feel Younger Program.

HOW A "PROTEIN PUNCH" HELPED PUT BETTY R. ON THE ROAD TO YOUTH

Betty R. was frail at birth. At a very early age, she succumbed to diphtheria which left her weak and frail. Lacking resistance, she contracted one infectious illness after another during her childhood. Bronchial disorders left her thin and wasted. Betty R. skipped so many of her daily classes that a private teacher had to be hired to help her at home. Most of the time Betty was either in bed or reclining on a couch. Her health was weak and she looked far older than she really was. She remained prematurely aged until her middle twenties. Then Betty R. found that Nature had a program that would help build her resistance to illness and help promote a look and feel of youth.

Gelatin Powder Helps Invigorate Metabolism. Betty R. was preparing a gelatin dish for herself when she discovered that the electricity had been turned off in her refrigerator. A local storm had cut off some of the power and she was left with a useless refrigerator. She looked at the bowl of dissolved gelatin powder and wondered whether to discard it (since it could not properly set without refrigeration) or to drink it as she had heard others do. Being thrifty, she decided to drink it. That was the start. From the beginning, she felt that the gelatin powder helped stimulate her sluggish metabolism. She began to feel better.

The electricity remained shut off for two days so Betty R. had to subsist on gelatin powder drinks and other fresh vegetable drinks. The vegetables would otherwise spoil so she decided to juice them. It was this program that revitalized her system. When she had the services of a working refrigerator and was able to cook on her electric stove, she found that food now became more palatable and that digestion was much improved. The raw juice program had fed a stream of nourishing amino acids throughout Betty's body and began the return to youthful health that made her look younger and feel better. She consulted with several nutritionists and came up with a special 3-ingredient liquid food that made her look and feel younger. Here is Betty's special liquid food:

Protein Punch

3 tablespoons of unflavored gelatin powder
1 whole banana
1 cup soy milk

Place the three ingredients in a blender. Whir for a few minutes until thoroughly blended. Drink slowly. This Protein Punch should be taken at least three times daily.

TEN BENEFITS OF THE PROTEIN PUNCH

Betty R. began her slow but steady return to youthful health on a special liquid food program that emphasized this Protein Punch. Here are the 10 benefits of this all-natural liquid food:

1. *Improves Blood Health.* Amino acids in the Protein Punch help nourish the hemoglobin which is 95 per cent protein.

2. *Resists Infection.* Amino acids help create antibodies which are needed to fight infection.

3. *Self-cleansing.* Amino acids feed the liver to enable it to help detoxify poisons and waste substances in the body.

4. *Heals Kidneys.* As a valuable filtering plant through which some 150 quarts of fluid pass daily, the kidneys require the amino acids in the Protein Punch which are speedily and "instantly" available for use.

5. *Controls Weight.* A swelling of body tissues caused by waterlogging may be traced to a protein deficiency. Amino acids in the Protein Punch help regulate the water balance of tissues and control weight.

6. *Body Repair.* Frequent bruises, cuts, and scratches need protein for healing. The Protein Punch helps promote this youthful ability for body repair.

7. *Energy Source.* Amino acids in the Protein Punch help nourish the muscles and promote a feeling of energy and vigor. Tired or flabby muscles create fatigue. Help strengthen muscle tissues with amino acids.

8. *Posture Improvement.* Amino acids send a stream of strength to the stomach and chest muscles and help keep them firm, improving posture.

9. *Feeds Skin, Hair, Fingernails.* All of these body parts depend upon amino acids. Betty R. enjoyed better skin color, thicker hair and less-brittle nails with her Protein Punch.

10. *Normal Regularity.* Amino acids help nourish intestinal muscles to transport food into the intestinal canal and promote normal regularity.

SPECIAL BENEFITS OF PROTEIN PUNCH: Betty R. found that the gelatin is a powerhouse of speedily assimilated protein.

The unique benefit of the banana is that its carbohydrates (highly digestible) perform a special protein-sparing action. This benefit is maximally effective when protein and carbohydrates are taken together in a live food juice such as the Protein Punch. The soy bean milk was rich in many valuable amino acids that created a soothing digestion. The combination of these *three* foods in liquid form helped promote an internal youth that reflected in Betty R.'s rejuvenation. She continued on this program, selected natural foods, eliminated artificial or prepared foods, and was soon so well recovered that she could work part-time in a nearby office. It is hoped that Nature will continue its improvement and that Betty R. can soon work full-time. She was able to drink her protein to a "Younger Feeling."

WHY SEED SPROUTS ARE NATURE'S PROTEIN-PLUS FOODS

Chewing difficulties compelled Laurence E. to consume large amounts of plant juices to help provide him with nutrients he ordinarily would pass up because he could not tackle a thick steak. Laurence E. was always pale, waxen in color, frequently losing days of work when he grew fatigued and contracted a virus. He took a brief vacation at a farm where he was given special seed sprouts. He discovered that seed sprouts are Nature's protein-plus foods because of a unique benefit to the body. Namely, the protein content of seeds is especially energized during sprouting and creates a dynamic invigoration in the system.

Laurence E. learned how to sprout seeds and made this special Seed Sprout Juice Tonic:

How To Sprout: Use clean, bright organic seeds. Select fenugreek, alfalfa, cress, radish, sunflower, pumpkin, wheat-rye, oats, corn, soybeans, black-eyed peas, lima beans, lentils, and parsley. Select them at any nearby seed merchant. Be sure to obtain *organically* grown seeds that are free of chemical pesticides and chemical sprays

Soak overnight in a wide mouth Mason jar. In the morning, drain and use this liquid for your special Sprout Juice Tonic. You may add a little sea salt to help increase the Tonic's mineral content.

Benefit: Sprouting increases the nutrition of the seed, powerhousing the protein content and developing an enzymatic action. Sprouted wheat has what is regarded the easiest-to-digest protein. These seed juices are a powerhouse of amino acids that work to nourish the entire system.

Eat the Sprouts: After you have consumed the protein-rich Sprout Juice Tonic, place the soaked seeds in the jar, cover the top with nylon tulle or stainless steel screen wire, cut to fit. Screw lid on tightly. Water under tap, two or three times a day. Turn on side in the bowl or pan to drain or set completely upside-down on two small boards to drain well. Eat these sprouts when the root is as long as the seed. Serve raw with a little honey and a sliced fruit for breakfast or dessert. Or, add to soups or salads just before serving. Chop into salads. Use in a Green Drink and chew the sprouts well after you have finished the Green Drink.

How Seed Sprout Juice Tonic Helped Laurence. This program did help Laurence with the following four benefits:

1. Seed sprout juice provides amino acids. These "building blocks" are the raw materials needed to create growth and repair of all body parts.

2. The Seed Sprout Juice Tonic gave Laurence a treasure of digestive enzymes that are youth-builders because they regulate metabolism and hormonal flow and influence all Look and Feel Young processes. The amino acids in the Tonic promoted this enzymatic flow in the digestive system.

3. The Seed Sprout Juice Tonic is a prime source of the amino acids that have a collodial osmotic pressure which helps make up blood proteins. These blood proteins then nourish the bloodstream, the rivers of youthful life. Laurence E. felt warmth in his extremities and looked glowingly youthful with an amino acid enriched bloodstream.

4. Laurence E. experienced welcome energy. The Seed Sprout Juice Tonic had a readily-available amino acid which

was changed into glucose and glycogen. In this form, it was stored in the liver to be used in situations where more energy was required. This helped promote youthful energy.

RECOVERY IS BRIEF. The problem here is that Laurence E. worked in a clothing store and would often work from morning until very late in the evening. He ate machine-prepared foods that were preserved, dehydrated, pre-heated, processed, and saturated in tissue-corroding chemical additives. He neglected his live food juice need and he soon felt a recurring decline in health. A mild heart seizure caused hospitalization. Recovery now seems doubtful. Laurence E. had his chance!

HOW A SPECIAL "AMINO COCKTAIL" PROMOTES A "LOOK ALIVE" FEELING

A condition of cirrhosis of the liver left Edna T. a semi-invalid. (It is believed that cirrhosis of the liver is traced to a partial nutritional deficiency and weakness of this organ to act as a filtering agent. This condition occurs when the normal functioning cells are replaced by harder, fibrous tissues, like scar tissues. Prolonged cirrhosis leads to the appearance of nail-like projections on the outer surface of the liver.) Edna T. was told to eat much fresh meat, with emphasis upon fresh liver. But she had a problem. *She did not like liver!*

Health Declines. Edna T. was unable to eat liver, and disliked other forms of meats which meant she was denying herself the valuable amino acid healing powers of these foods. Her health declined. She found food, in general, to be unpalatable. Edna T. was soon confined to her bed.

Overhears Radio Lecture. The radio was her only source of diversion while she lay weak and spent in bed. She tuned in an early morning discussion show and heard a physician recommend a food called *desiccated liver*. The physician said that this was a dehydrated form of liver in which the fat and connective tissues were removed. In this powdered form, the liver was a powerhouse of vitamins minerals and most important of all, of minerals! A special dehydrating process preserved the protein–amino acid supply. The doctor said that this desiccated liver powder, mixed with tomato juice, forms a "binding action" with vitamins in the tomato juice and when sipped slowly, helps send a stream of organ-building amino acids into the system. It was the most effective substitute for whole liver that the doctor knew of.

Edna T. Prepares Special Protein Food. Edna decided to try this liver-substitute. She called all over town but was unable to locate a source. She finally found a local health food store and ordered a package of desiccated liver powder. She prepared a special health beverage which she called a Super-Plus Protein Booster because of its benefits.

Edna mixed two tablespoons of desiccated liver powder into one glass of tomato juice. She added a little lemon juice for a piquant flavor, stirring vigorously. She drank one glass in the morning, another glass at noon, a third glass in the evening.

Further Nutritional Improvements. At the start, the Super-Plus Protein Booster offered just a feeling of relaxation. Later, it helped stimulate her taste buds and she could partake of wholesome foods which included small broiled meat slices, fish, baked chicken, clear soups and broths Gradually, her strength returned. She continued to take the Super-Plus Protein Booster.

Enjoys Youthful Feeling. Several months of special protein boosting foods helped Edna out of her bed. She felt youthful, her face looked colorful and her grip was stronger. She could do housework with enthusiasm and not drudgery. Of course, her complete health was not restored because the prolonged disorder had left her wasted. But she had a youthful attitude and this made her feel well enough to be able to take a part-time job. She continues with her daily Super-Plus Protein Booster as Nature's own "youth insurance."

BENEFITS OF SUPER-PLUS PROTEIN BOOSTER: The tonic or liquid form of this food juice means that you are given a pre-digested form of health-building amino acids. Ordinarily, when you eat protein, your digestive tract must split it into amino acids to pass it through the membrane walls of the alimentary canal. In conditions of weakness or poor digestive ability, this is not always possible. A congested alimentary tract has an accumulation of decomposed protein. Some may be forced through, but the rest remains as a stumbling block to complete internal youth. A Super-Plus Protein Booster means that the amino acids are pre-digested in the tomato juice through its mineral action and you are actually *drinking amino acids!* This is the unique benefit offered by Nature in the form of these juices.

How the Super-Plus Protein Booster Provides "Younger Feeling" Amino Acids. This powerful booster offers your system these "Younger Feeling" amino acids: *Valine* helps spark mental vigor, muscular coordination, and smooth nerve health. *Lysine* influences body growth factors, nourishes the bloodstream, forms antibodies, and improves eyesight. *Tryptophane* works to nourish the skin and hair, metabolize the B-complex vitamin group, improve digestion and nervous system. *Methionine* is sent to the liver and kidneys to regenerate the cells. *Cystine* supplies over 10 per cent of the insulin needed by your pancreas for assimilation of sugars and starches. *Phenylaline* is food for your thyroid glands to secrete a hormone to promote emotional health. *Arginine* helps detoxify poisonous wastes and filter out toxic substances. *Glutamic acid* boosts emotional health by entering into the delicate functions of the brain. *Histidine* stimulates and feeds the auditory nerve needed for good hearing; many nerve cells of the hearing mechanisms need this valuable amino acid. *Threonine* helps the digestive and intestinal tracts to function smoothly; this amino acid also helps extract nutrients and speed them into bodily assimilation and absorption.

Use the Super-Plus Protein Booster at One Special Time Each Day. In order to enable the amino acids to assimilate easier, this Super-Plus Protein Booster should be taken in the early afternoon when the luncheon meal is largely digested and the dinnertime meal is a while away. This enables nutrients in the desiccated liver tomato juice, and lemon juice to work together, combine and become more fully assimilated into the lymph and bloodstream *without* delay from the presence of other nutrients. Just one glass in the early afternoon will help give your digestion the working materials with which to promote the look and feel of youth. Amino acids *do* make a difference when they're in liquid food form!

All of you is protein. Without this miracle food, there might not be much of you! Nature meant for you to enjoy prolonged life and youth through the power of amino acids. Drink your way to everlasting benefits with live food juices.

IN REVIEW:

1. Amino acids are vital in promoting the look and feel of youth. In the form of live food juices, they have three special outlined benefits.

2. A special "Protein Punch" put Betty R. back on the road to youth. Make it yourself, using three "magic amino acid" foods. It offers ten outlined youth restorative benefits.

3. Seed sprouts are Nature's own protein-plus foods. Make a Seed Sprout Juice Tonic and enjoy health rejuvenation as did Laurence E.

4. A special "Amino Cocktail" promotes the yearned-for "Look Alive" feeling. Just two ingredients can make all the difference in the world of health.

5. A Super-Plus Protein Booster promotes well-being and a feeling of "glad-to-be-alive."

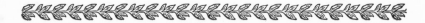

Chapter 9

How to Create Healing Sleep

for Youthfulness through

Special Liquid Foods

A good night's sleep may well be considered Nature's perfect health and youth tonic. If sleep could be made into a tonic, it certainly would help ease many of the ills faced by people with various disturbances. In the form of special liquid foods, sleep *can* become a special tonic, so to speak.

THE VITAMIN GROUP THAT PROMOTES RESTFUL SLEEP

The B-complex group of vitamins is known for containing ingredients that help bring about an internal oxidative process that lends itself to a natural form of sleep. These "sleep inducing" vitamins play a decisive role in the oxidative process that goes on in each body cell. They are part of the enzymes which help carbohydrates become metabolized.

Nervous tissue is *relaxed* when this carbohydrate oxidation process is accomplished.

Sources of B-Complex Vitamins. Brewer's yeast powder, soy bean powder, sunflower seed oil, and wheat germ powder represent powerful supplies of this all-essential nutrient. Using these powders and oils, you can create a healthful tonic to create a desire for sleep.

NATURE'S OWN NIGHT CAP. Here is how to make a sleep tonic that is all-natural and works to promote a nerve relaxation that induces sleep.

Mix together one tablespoon of brewer's yeast powder, soy bean powder, and wheat germ flakes. Add freshly poured water and stir vigorously (a blender is best). Add two tablespoons of sunflower seed oil. Drink about one hour before going to sleep.

Benefits: The combination of B-complex vitamins works to soothe frazzled nerves, helps to draw away "tension pockets" through liberating "kinks" in the circulatory network, and promotes a relaxation that is conducive to sleep.

HOW STEPHEN R. USES NATURE FOR A SLEEPING POTION. Stephen R. is an overworked sales executive for a leading department store chain. He has many family financial obligations, not to mention responsibilities for his company. He is too conscientious in his effort to succeed, but you just cannot convince Stephen of that. He tosses and turns nightly because he takes his business problems to bed with him. His energy level was getting lower. He began to show symptoms of premature and unnecessary aging. Prolonged insomnia made him severely nervous and irritable. He snapped at buyers and was sharply rebuked by his superiors who sensed a breakdown. He almost lost the position he labored so hard to build up.

European Executive Shows Him How to Use a Nature Tonic to Stimulate Healthful Sleep. His condition was noted by a visiting European executive who inquired about Stephen's health. Stephen said he tried hard to sleep but it didn't come. The executive said that was his mistake. You just cannot order yourself to sleep. You cannot drive yourself to sleep as you drive yourself to work! You have to welcome sleep by means of Nature. The executive said he had worked among Orientals and noticed they were always calm and relaxed. One Oriental businessman said that it was a tradition to have a special sleeping tonic—all natural—about one hour before turning in. The executive suggested it to Stephen who tried it. Here is how it is made:

Oriental Sleeping Tonic

    1 cup milk (whole or skim)
    2 tablespoons rice polish (available at health stores)
    1 tablespoon natural honey
    1 tablespoon powdered skim milk
    1 teaspoon carob powder (available at health stores)

Pour one half the milk into a blender. Add all remaining ingredients. Mix thoroughly. Add remaining one half cup milk and mix a few seconds longer. Sip slowly.

Special Benefit: The powerful supply of calcium helps promote a relaxed heart, improve blood tone, and stabilize the blood pressure. The rice is a prime source of 100% digested amlyopectin—a special nutrient that promotes a youthful circulatory system. The honey contains minerals that ease internal pressures and the other ingredients work harmoniously to soothe the entire nervous system.

Stephen R. Enjoys Partial Sleep. Using this Oriental Sleeping Tonic, Stephen R. did enjoy partial sleep. But his business pressures were so great that he only had a half night's sleep and could not obtain full benefits from this special tonic. However, he was less irritable so some progress was made. Live food juices can work if they form part of a *complete* program of health restoration. The *complete* program calls for natural foods and a work-play-recreation-rest balance. Everything in moderation. Abuse yourself and you receive only partial restoration of health. It is hoped that Stephen will follow the other natural laws of healthful living to promote the look and feel of youth.

HOW WARM LIQUIDS HELP PROMOTE
YOUTHFUL SLEEP

Jenny T. lives in a warm climate that makes her thirsty all the time. She imbibes much soda pop soft drinks. The problem here is that most carbonated soft drinks contain caffeine, a substance that activates the adrenal cortex and causes excessive stimulation. Both the ice cold drinks which are stimulants and the internal chilling that works against the feeling of relaxation cheated her of youthful sleep. Jenny T. was actually "aging" herself by "soda pop insomnia."

Changes to Herb Teas. When a doctor put her on a no-caffeine program, she had to give up soda drinks. She also eliminated coffee. As for tea, she never liked conventional tea. However, in a folk recipe, she read of herb tea so she purchased some. She found that it promoted a youthful feeling of joy to her middle region which promoted a desire for sleep. Now she could enjoy a youthful sleep. Refreshing sleep is able to give you energy and vigor to rival that of a youngster! Now Jenny T. looked and felt better. Even though the weather was hot, she learned that a cup of freshly brewed herb tea could make her relax her way to youthful sleep.

Herb teas are sold at almost all health stores; available in tea bag or loose form, depending upon your desire, they should be a nightly custom to help induce the sandman.

WHY CALCIUM IS A NATURAL SLEEP TONIC. As a mineral, calcium helps promote a soothing alkaline-acid balance in the bloodstream and thereby promote a smooth resilient circulatory system. A folk remedy is one that calls for the following calcium tonic that might well be regarded as:

Nu-Youth Sleep Tonic

2 whole bananas
1 cup skim milk or soy milk
2 tablespoons honey

Put peeled bananas into a blender, add the milk and honey. Whir vigorously until assimilated. Drink one hour before bedtime.

Benefit of Nu-Youth Sleep Tonic: The milk calcium is blended into the nitrogen-phosphorus-calcium-minerals of the banana to form a special "retention" power. This means that it has a satiety value in its speedy assimilation into the bloodstream to promote an overall relaxation. When you enjoy a youthful sleep with the Nu-Youth Sleep Tonic, you begin to look and feel younger! The banana is also a reliable source of vitamins A, B-complex, niacin, essential minerals, amino acids, and Vitamin C. When added to milk with its "almost perfect" supply of nearly all natural elements, you have created a live food juice that is brimming with elements to create a healthful relaxation. *Extra-Special Benefit:* the bananas, milk and honey are Nature's foods—made by Nature. Surely you should want to obtain a healthful sleeping tonic from Nature instead of from a chemical laboratory!

THE FARMER'S BRAN BROTH

Rosa E. found city life too strenuous. She looked worn, wan and haggard. She fled to a farm for a little vacation but found her nerves so tense that she could scarcely sleep. Rosa E. lamented over having spent so much money for this farm vacation with the hopes of being able to sleep, and here she was, tossing and turning, listening to the rustle of the wind in the treetops and the sounds of barnyard fowl and unable to relax. She might have continued on with her chronic insomnia had not the farmer's wife mentioned overhearing her tossing and turning.

Farmer's Wife Suggests Folk Brew. The farmer's wife listened to Rosa's tearful plea to be able to sleep. Then she said there were times when even farmers and so-called country folks also had insomnia. She suggested the following:

Bran Sleep Broth

1 cup bran (from red wheat, if possible)
2 cups water

To make: Early afternoon, soak the bran in water. Early evening, pour into strainer and drain. Pour 1 cup hot water through the bran, stirring thoroughly, rinsing as much as possible. Add 1 cup hot water and sip slowly, about an hour before bedtime.

Special Benefits: The rich supply of nerve-calming calcium and the combined B-complex vitamins unite with the amino acids to create an overall feeling of natural tranquility throughout the circulatory system. The comfortably hot broth also gives a gentle relaxation to the tense vascular network.

Rosa E. Unable to Sleep at First. Because she was so wrought up, Rosa E. could not sleep at first. It took a few evenings of Bran Sleep Broth before she could be sufficiently relaxed to be able to sleep. She took the recipe back home with her and she will probably be able to discard her tranquilizers in favor of Nature.

WHY THE BRAN SLEEP BROTH PROMOTES A YOUTHFUL SLEEP. Here are some benefits of the Bran Sleep Broth. The ingested nutrients perform the following youth restorative sleep benefits:

1. Nutrients help stabilize breathing.

2. The heart is kept at a tranquil and normal beat.

3. Body temperature is stabilized so that pressure is more regulated.

4. Body processes (digestion, assimilation, circulation, respiration) are relaxed, refreshed, and rejuvenated through healing sleep.

5. The brain is renourished; the pattern of brain waves may change, but the waves become more stabilized and relaxed.

6. As the sleeping period approaches its end, the nutrients now help the temperature, respiration, pulse and blood pressure become adjusted to waking activities.

7. Awakening, the sleep cycle is ended and there is a

feeling of renewed and refreshed energy that promotes the look and energy of youth.

The farmer's Bran Sleep Broth, in combination with healthful living programs, can help to promote a youthful sleep.

HOW TO CREATE A FAVORABLE SLEEPING ENVIRONMENT

A health tonic offers the start of the sleep cycle. But favorable surroundings help to spur on the sleep. The arrangement of your bedroom and the condition of the bed itself affect your sleep more than you might think. If your nights have been wakeful, give a thought to your surroundings. When you go to bed, look about you critically for anything that could disturb your sleep.

Glare Is Disturbing. Do street lights glare at you? Are they reflected about the room from mirrors or shiny metal objects? Does the woodwork have a high, glossy finish? Are window shades or draperies transparent? Is the bed in the darkest part of the room? These are conditions that should be remedied.

Other Suggestions: If street lights are bothersome, block them off with a folding screen; even a high-backed chair will help a lot. Mirrors or other shiny surfaces that reflect light can either be draped or moved to other positions. Dark green window shades are better than light-colored semi-transparent ones. When your room is to be done over, try flat paints or soft colors, quiet wallpaper and dark rugs to absorb rather than reflect light. Your aim should be to make your bedroom a restful place, not a loud one.

Special Aids. If after doing these things, your room is still too light, then try an eye mask. Black, soft-textured cloth will do or you can buy a ready-made one at the pharmacy or a health food store. When morning light is the only nuisance, you can train yourself to don the mask almost automatically if it is kept beside the bed. Nurses and sanatorium patients who must sleep during the day have proved that these aids are beneficial for daytime sleeping. They should be doubly beneficial for night time sleeping.

For restful sleep, your bed should maintain your body in a straight line and should have soft, light fluffy blankets.

NATURAL SLEEPING METHODS

Proper Bed. A coil (box) spring comes nearest to maintaining your backbone in a straight line because each individual coil "gives" according to the weight directly over it. As a substitute, the so-called link spring, made of jointed wire links with strong springs at head and foot, will probably be better than the woven wire or fabric spring which tends to sag like a hammock. People with spinal or sacroiliac disturbances should have medical advice for the spring and mattress best suited for them.

Good Mattress. Is your mattress free of lumps and hollows? In inner-spring mattresses, the top and bottom padding tends to be pressed into lumps from long usage and should be renovated or replaced. In cold weather, inner-spring mattresses may prove too cool unless a blanket is placed between springs and mattress.

Pillow Talk. When your pillow is of proper thickness, it helps to keep the head in a straight line with the spine. Pillows are sold in varying thicknesses to suit individual needs.

Blankets. Blankets that are soft and fluffy conserve body warmth without adding the extra weight that interferes with sleep. Modern, electric blankets are fine from this standpoint, and because they are thermostatically controlled; a single blanket does the job in any weather. Keep you feet warm to induce a healthful desire to sleep.

NATURE VS. DRUGS. A habit-forming sleeping pill leaves the insomniac "doped" during the day, which only adds to the youth-robbing misery. There are also risks. Drugs often lead to a trance-like state instead of sleep. An overdose may often lead to death. Nature, on the other hand, works to correct the *cause* of insomnia, not just the symptoms as is in the case of drugs. Look to Nature to help promote sound, refreshing sleep and self-rejuvenation.

SUMMARY:

1. Vitamin B-complex group in a tonic relaxes the nerves through a carbohydrate oxidation process to induce natural sleep.
2. The Nature's Own Night Cap is reportedly soothing to promote youthful sleep. All-natural!
3. Stephen R. found blessed sleep through the Oriental Sleeping Tonic.
4. Warm liquids are more sleep-inducing than ice cold caffeine-containing cola drinks.
5. Nu-Youth Sleep Tonic has unique vitamin-mineral benefits to promote healthful sleep.
6. The farmer's Bran Sleep Broth is a folk potion that has special Look and Feel Younger benefits.
7. Create a favorable sleeping environment by eliminating glare, using an eye mask, having a proper bed, mattress, pillow and blanket.
8. Grow young through restful-rejuvenating sleep—without drugs.

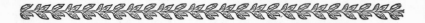

Chapter 10

How Programmed "Water

Drinking" Can Ease

Digestive-Nerve Disorders

for Dynamic Youthfulness

THE famed spa baths of the ancients helped promote a well-lubricated digestive-nerve health that gave a look and feel of dynamic youthfulness. The ancients were well aware of the soothing comfort and overall refreshment made possible by regular bathing and fresh water drinking. The spa baths were sites of youthful replenishment through controlled water drinking.

HOW WATER BECOMES A "YOUTH TONIC" IN THE DIGESTIVE SYSTEM

Fresh water is Nature's own "youth tonic" when it is introduced into the body. Here are some of the benefits of programmed water drinking as they relate to your digestive and nerve system:

Helps Wash Insides. When you drink a glass of water, it goes to your stomach. Part of it is absorbed directly into the bloodstream through the walls of your stomach. The rest of the water goes to your intestines where it helps to keep the food in a liquid state while it is being absorbed. This, too, is then absorbed into your bloodstream. For a few moments after you drink water, your blood is somewhat "washed" as it is thinned; after that, the liquids are speedily distributed to other parts of your body for youthful moisturization.

Water Facilitates Digestion. Water is continually shifting about the body to provide a vehicle for digestive juices and other secretions, to transport nutriments and carry off waste products. Equilibrium within narrow limits is maintained between circulating fluids, extracellular and intracellular, free and bound water. Adjustments can be made very rapidly.

Helps Refresh and Maintain a Youthful Bloodstream. The fluid inside the cells and outside the cells of the body is continually being shifted and moved. The fluid conveys every substance that moves from place to place. Water enables *absorption, diffusion* and *secretion* to occur. Water also enters into the many chemical reactions in your body. The lymph is that fluid which circulates through the lymph glands as the blood circulates through blood vessels. Lymph apparently moves quite speedily from one part of your body to another and water is needed to promote this youthful function.

HOW WATER REJUVENATES YOUR BODY

Water is an essential constituent of living protoplasm. No cell functions when it is absolutely dry and most cells must be constantly bathed in fluid in order to remain youthfully healthy. Furthermore, your cells depend upon having their food transported to them over a fluid route (the blood), a demand which alone requires ten pounds of water to be in circulation constantly. Waste-bearing water (urine) is necessary to flush away the end products of metabolism. And without water to moisten the surface of the lungs, there can be no intake of oxygen or expulsion of carbon dioxide.

WATER SOOTHES YOUR NERVOUS SYSTEM. The nerve network is constantly in need of flexible lubricating materials such as water in order to keep them functioning in a smooth working condition. We all know how tempers become short during hot seasonal spells, and how the nerves become ragged when subjected to prolonged dehydration. A drink of fresh water helps moisten the delicate neuron cells and promote a youthful disposition and a better emotional attitude.

WATER: RIVER OF LIFE. Water is the vehicle for food materials absorbed from the digestive canal. It is the medium in which chemical changes take place that underlie most of our youth-creating activities. Water is essential in the regulation of body temperature and it plays an important role in mechanical surfaces such as the lubrication of the joints.

HOW NORMAN C. BOOSTED YOUTHFUL DIGESTION WITH PROGRAMMED WATER DRINKING

Norman C. found his digestion acting like a bottleneck in his stomach. He felt a heavy leaden weight after each meal which made him grouchy, nervous and easily upset. The accumulated partially digested "lumps" in his stomach gave him a stooped, bent over posture. He also felt so bloated that he developed a paunch and had to let his belt out a few more notches. Norman C. looked and felt much older than his 33 years.

Worsens Digestive Problem with Water Binge. Thinking his problem could be caused by lack of water (he hardly consumed much) he started bolting down glasses of water with his meal. But this only caused a water logging of his tissues, bloating of the system, and a "drowned" digestion. He had so loaded up his digestive tract with water that food became saturated like a sponge and remained insoluble and lumpy. He felt worse than before.

Corrects Schedule to Regular Water Drinking. It was this

trial and error mishap that led to Norman's eventual improvement of bloated digestion. He found that if he would drink up to two glasses of freshly poured tap water *in between meals,* approximately two hours either before or after lunch and dinner, then his digestion would be improved. He followed this program for three weeks and experienced relief from the pounding pressure of his accumulated digestive bulk. He then enjoyed better digestive power through water drinking on a regular schedule. His disposition improved. He felt lightheaded, happy, and youthful! Water had made him young again!

BENEFITS OF PROGRAMMED WATER DRINKING. If you follow this simple, all-natural schedule of drinking up to two glasses of water approximately two hours either *before* or *after* lunch and dinner, the process enables food to become properly digested, absorbed, and carried to all parts of the body via the bloodstream.

The Hydrolysis Benefit. This program promotes the look and feel of a young digestion through the process of *hydrolysis*—the reaction of food elements with water. This permits the reaction of water with proteins, starches, vitamins, sugars, and fats to produce substances which the body cells can use in their youth-building functions. Programmed water drinking permits the hydrolysis process to stimulate the gastric glands to facilitate digestion; furthermore, in the intestine, the moisturizing of solid food by the available water facilitates absorption of nutrients and the excretion of waste. *Hydrolysis is the youthful biological rhythm of healthful internal nourishment.*

Water Promotes Youthful Assimilation. The secret of youthful assimilation may be in the first step in the digestive process; namely, in the mouth where saliva (99$^{1}/_{2}$% water) starts the breakdown of carbohydrates. Water then transports the main proteins into the stomach where they are broken down and digested by watery gastric juices to create amino acids. From here the food, now in a comparatively fluid state, enters the upper section of the small intestine, known as the duodenum.

Water and a Young Digestive Tract. The enzymatic secretions of the duodenal wall itself, as well as the liver and pancreas (90% water) complete the digestive tract. The food then sails on watery lakes through other sections of the small intestine, into the large intestine or colon, and from there into the rectum.

Water is absorbed into the body throughout the digestive process; somewhat less absorption takes place in the upper portion of the digestive system than in the lower. But you do need ample liquids to help promote a smooth-functioning youthful digestive system.

REGULATE YOUR WATER INTAKE. It has been estimated that three and one-half to five and one-half quarts of water are used by the body daily in the digestive process; about a quart and a half of saliva, one or two quarts in the gastric juices, and the same amount in bile and other secretions. A substantial portion of this is reabsorbed through the intestinal wall to be used in carrying nutritive substances to the body. Water is also vital to the excretion of soluble wastes through the lungs. It is estimated that you need up to eight glasses of water daily. If you regulate or program your intake to having *two glasses in between meals,* you will be helping to maintain a youthful digestive quality.

HOW WATER CORRECTED ELSIE'S ALLERGIC DISTRESS

Elsie W. was a librarian. She also worked part-time doing statistical research for a large manufacturing plant. This put her in contact with so many musty, dusty books and papers as well as endless files that it left her with an allergic disorder.

Elsie developed a form of asthmatic-bronchial distress that left her coughing, sneezing, and wheezing whenever she came in contact with dusty papers. She had to give up her part-time job and was in jeopardy of losing her librarian job. She corrected her food intake to emphasize natural, wholesome, and additive-free foods and while she experienced partial relief, she still felt "sandy" in her throat, "grains" in her nose, and "burning sensation" in her eyes when she had to handle papers and books. For a while Elsie W. thought she might become a victim of chronic bronchial distress.

New Office Water Cooler Helps Elsie W. An office renovation program meant that the library would be able to have a water cooler in Elsie's private cubicle. Now she would be able to drink water. It was this event that gave her relief from her bronchial distress. Elsie found that her symptoms became eased. She had started to drink water regularly and this promoted a youthful respiratory tract. After several months, she was much improved; her allergic distress vanished and she was re-hired by the statistical company at a slight increase in salary. Water made her young again!

How Water Improved Elsie's Allergic Resistance. The walls of the tiny air sacs that make up the lungs must be moistened continuously so that oxygen can enter the body and carbon dioxide be expelled. Not only the lungs, but the nose, throat, trachea, and bronchial branches of the respiratory tract are coated with fluid. By drinking up to four glasses of water daily, Elsie W. moistened this delicate region, gave her organs a youthful moisture and was able to resist and correct her allergic problems.

WATER KEEPS A HEALTHY KIDNEY CONDITION. Under normal conditions of temperature and activity, the kidneys are the principal avenue of water elimination. The amount varies with the amount of water intake. Generally, one quart of water passing through the kidneys will carry with it one and one-half ounces of soluble waste. In the normal adult, the amount of urine varies with fluid intake; it can be reduced through perspiration. During metabolic activity, wastes are produced which must be excreted through the kidneys. A fresh available water supply helps promote this kidney-excretion function to keep the entire body washed and cleansed. Water helps to maintain a healthy kidney condition.

WATER MAINTAINS FIRM MUSCLE TONUS. Gerald T. was troubled with sagging muscles. At age 42, he had always been proud of his firm body. Now, his arms showed sagging skin, his muscles looked "drooped" and his entire body started to have a ptosis (dropped) slump. Gerald T. tried exercises but these caused such a rapid evaporation of moisture that he became dehydrated. He envied other businessmen at a special health club for their firm muscle tonus. He did not share their belief that fresh water and liquid foods could help "nourish" muscle tissues and keep them firm. He soon developed crepe-like skin and was embarrassed to appear on the beach or to wear short-sleeved shirts. His sagging chin was the start of his decline in age. All this at just 42. If he had heeded the suggestions of the others and used liquid foods and water, he might have grown younger as did the others!

Water Nourishes Muscles. The muscles, which are 75 per cent water, must have liquids to contract and maintain proper and youthful tonus. Good water-nourished muscle tone helps serve to protect the body. Water serves to lubricate the joints and muscles and act as a cushion to protect the body from injuries resulting from impact and shock. Water makes it possible for organs within muscle parts to slide smoothly. Water also serves to stabilize pressure in muscular parts of the body, such as the eyeballs.

SET A WATER PROGRAMMING SCHEDULE. The simplest way to help promote a youthful water-sufficient body is to develop a drinking pattern that becomes as automatic and irrevocable a habit as brushing the teeth. It is sensible to program your water drinking *between* meals at set hours; vary the hours if you change your meal schedules.

For some people, drinking a small amount of liquid with meals will help promote the secretion and activity of the digestive juices and absorption of the ingested food. It also helps retard the growth of intestinal bacteria and lessen the extent of putrefactive processes in the intestine.

HOW TO TEST YOUR OWN WATER NEED. It has been noted that when the body's urine is acid, then the water supply is about average. You can test any possible water deficiency, with your doctor's approval, by this simple method:

At any pharmacy, purchase Squibb-Nitrazine paper (or

similar product). Dip a small corner of this paper in your urine sample. A chart on the container of the Nitrazine paper will provide explicit instructions; or ask the pharmacist and your doctor. If the paper is yellow, your urine is normal and acid. If the paper shows another color, it means that your urine is too alkaline. Discuss it with your physician.

HOME WATER TONIC. Since acid is the natural condition of the urine, it is youthfully beneficial to keep it that way. Acidic urine means that your kidneys are doing a youthfully efficient job of washing out body wastes and impurities. To help keep the kidneys in good condition, try this Home Water Tonic:

Mix together one average glass (6 ounces) of water with two tablespoons of natural apple cider vinegar. Mix thoroughly and drink the first thing in the morning. Minerals in the apple cider vinegar form a binding action to ingredients in the water and help keep the condition of the urine in its beneficial acid state.

YOUTHFUL ENERGY WITH A "WATER" BREAK. Fatigue can be transformed into youthful energy with a "water break." This was shown to be so by researchers at a large company. They found that worker energy could be made more youthful by having a "water break" twice a day—fifteen minutes for each break—one at 9:30 in the morning just before the curve took its sharpest dip; the second "water break" at 2:30 in the afternoon, the lowest point of the after-lunch period. Just one glass at each of these times reportedly promoted digestive-nerve invigoration and a youthful feeling of energy. Fatigue is often traced to a lowering of the body's fluid balance—so take a "water break" and *drink yourself to youthful energy!*

WATER: NATURE'S YOUTH POTION. Nearly all vital youth-promoting processes are in need of liquid refreshment. Even the bones have up to 20% water. We know that water holds in suspension, or solution, the nutrients needed to sustain youth; water dissolves such gases as oxygen and carbon dioxide as well as proteins, minerals, vitamins, hormones, and enzymes. The digestive process, being a chemical reaction, must be facilitated by water to hold the enzymes in solution and hasten the reaction of digestion. The digested materials must then be put in solution before they can be used to promote the look and feel of youth.

Water further distributes youthful warmth and heat throughout the entire body. Water acts in the body's cooling system by its rapid circulation in the blood; it also dissipates unnecessary heat through the agency of perspiration and its evaporation. Water moistens the lungs. Water lubricates the heart, intestines, and other organs so they may move without abrasive friction. Joints are in need of being lubricated with water in the synovial fluids. If these fluids "dry out," there is a stiffening-aging of the muscles and joints. Water enters into most body processes and contributes to the five senses of speech, sight, hearing, smell, and taste. *Water is youthful life!*

HIGHLIGHTS OF CHAPTER IO:

1. Fresh water is Nature's own youth tonic. Drink regularly. Obtain bottled spring water wherever possible.
2. Water rejuvenates digestion, refreshes the bloodstream, and promotes an overall nerve-digestive improvement.
3. Norman C. boosted youthful digestion with a simple-to-follow water drinking program.
4. The hydrolysis benefit of water drinking helps promote the look and feel of a young digestion.
5. A special water drinking program helped correct Elsie W.'s allergic distress.
6. Water helps nourish muscles to keep them firm and youthful.
7. Test your own water need with the Nitrazine paper method.
8. Create youthful energy with a "water" break.

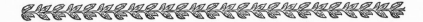

Chapter 11

How to Use Natural Raw Juices for Your Youthful Heart's Benefit

AN all-natural seed juice, available at almost all health stores as well as many supermarkets, has been seen to produce remarkably effective rejuvenation upon the heart. This seed juice, in combination with several all-natural vegetable juices, serves to promote a healthful oxygenation to the heart, stimulate the circulation if it is sluggish, and give a look and feel of youth to the entire body. These natural raw juices are valuable for their rejuvenation benefits to the mind and body. They are available at modest cost. The reward? A lifetime of improved vitality when used together with other natural laws of youthful living.

THE DYNAMIC HEALTH POWER OF SEED JUICE. Wheat germ oil is known for being a dynamic source of Vitamin E, the miracle "youth vitamin" for the heart. Vitamin E is an oil-soluble nutrient found in the oils of the wheat germ and other seed plants. It is found in leafy vegetables and other plants as well. It is present in different amounts in your body's tissues; it is more concentrated in fatty tissues and such internal organs as the liver and heart. It serves a basic function to help nourish, repair, replenish, and sustain the trillions of body cells to promote the look and feel of youth. In particular, Vitamin E, as a seed juice in the form of wheat germ oil, when combined with Vitamins B-complex and C, helps invigorate the heart muscle with amazing benefits.

HEART HEALTH JUICE

Bernice E. was able to strengthen her heart when put on a special corrective food program emphasizing Vitamins B-complex, C, and E. She then prepared a special Heart Health Juice consisting of the following nutrient-rich foods:

> ½ cup tomato juice
> 1 tablespoon brewer's yeast powder
> ½ cup seasonal citrus juice
> 6 tablespoons cold-pressed wheat germ oil

Stir vigorously or mix in a blender. Drink one glass during early morning, another glass several hours after lunch, a final glass several hours after dinner.

Bernice E. was using these natural raw juices to help strengthen the vascular-circulatory system and improve her heart health. After several months of improved living customs with emphasis upon natural foods, and with the above Heart Health Juice, thrice daily, she was greatly improved—she had roses in her cheeks, her hands were steady, her memory improved. She continues this Heart Health Juice daily as part of her program to enjoy the look and feel of youth.

FOUR "HEART-HEALING" BENEFITS OF HEART HEALTH JUICE. The "secret" here is in Vitamin E, the miracle seed juice that works with the other nutrients to perform the following benefits to the heart:

. *Revitalizes Bloodstream.* Vitamin E is known to be a natural anti-thrombin (dissolves bloodclots) in the bloodstream. It was found that Vitamin E was a substance normally circulating in the blood of all young persons to help reduce clot occurrence. It is an all-natural substance that helps accelerate external healing and also prevents internal clotting situations.

2. *Provides Healthful Internal Oxygen.* Vitamin E, with the other nutrients, performs the youth-giving function of internal oxygen conservation. Vitamin E is a natural anti-oxidant in the body. It has been shown to decrease the oxygen requirement of muscle by as much as 43 per cent; it creates a narrow stream of blood which gets through the narrowed coronary artery in many heart patients. This helps reduce the occurrence of anoxia (lack of oxygen) which is the trigger that sets off anginal or heart pain.

3. *Melts Unwanted Internal Scar Tissue.* Vitamin E serves the major heart youth function in preventing internal scar tissue production; in some reported instances, it helps bring about a melting of unwanted scars. It also helps stimulate circulation to favor overall young heart health.

4. *Helps Dilate Blood Vessels.* Vitamin E is a dilator of blood vessels. This was demonstrated by X-rays in tests by doctors. It helps open up new pathways in the aging circulation, and spares blocks produced by clots and hardened arteries.

It's All Natural. Vitamin E with the other listed ingredients creates an all-natural raw juice that is free from drugs and medications. This makes it especially beneficial for the youth-seeker who cannot tolerate drugs.

RAW JUICE COCKTAIL GIVES "SECOND" LIFE

A 72-year-old man is reported to have found a second life through the use of two nutrients. These are both Vitamin C and E that can be mixed together as a Raw Juice Heart Cocktail. Mix one glass of freshly squeezed orange juice with five tablespoons of any seed oil. Wheat germ oil is especially beneficial for its high Vitamin E content. The 72-year-old man said that he had had a serious auto accident. His chest was injured but no bones were broken which was fortunate. Jack M. was examined by doctors and X-rays showed that his heart muscles were damaged. The doctors gave him medication but it only made Jack M. feel worse. *Tries Raw Juice Heart Cocktail.* He took the combination of Vitamin C and E and found that his breathing became normal, his chest pains went away and he could perform normal activities with no strain. At 72, Jack M. was younger than others half his age! The Raw Juice Heart Cocktail gave him a "second" youth.

GRACE J. FEELS YOUNG AT 57. The power of raw juices with emphasis upon a seed oil with Vitamin E was reported by a physician with regard to Grace J. At age 57, she suffered the clutching pains of angina when she strained herself. Under examination, 57-year old Grace showed ulcers of the duodenal or small intestine. A cardiogram indicated a coronary artery disease.

Heart-Youth Tonic Promotes Youth. A special tonic was prepared in which ten tablespoons of cold-pressed wheat germ oil was mixed into a glass of freshly squeezed lettuce juice. Daily, Grace J. took this Heart-Youth Tonic. Within six months, it is reported that Grace J. was free of all chest pain. She was even able to swim a quarter of a mile! The interesting point here is that few "young and healthy" persons—and those younger than 57—can swim a quarter mile without some exhaustion. But Grace did it and she felt younger than young at 57. She still takes this Heart-Youth Tonic daily and is rewarded with the look and feel of youth-*plus!*

WHY SEED AND FOOD JUICES SHOULD BE COMBINED. To help keep your heart young and healthy, seek a balance. It is noted that Vitamin E protects the body's store of other vitamins, especially Vitamin A and C found in almost all raw fruits and vegetables. Both Vitamins A and C are sensitive to the presence of oxygen and may lose much of their youth-giving benefits over a period of time.

With the presence of Vitamin E in the digestive tract, these vitamins are protected from oxidation. Hence the heart-benefit of mixing together seed oil with desired fresh raw fruit and/or vegetable juices. A *blend* of Vitamins A, C and E produces this unique hidden youth factor. The three ingredients work together to maintain the purity and availability of oxygen in the system.

RAW JUICE HEART TRANQUILIZER. A youthful heart is one that is well nourished with nutrients found in this Raw Juice Heart Tranquilizer. It contains substances that are worked into the bloodstream and promote an alert hormonal system.

> 10 tablespoons wheat germ oil
> 1/2 cup carrot juice
> 1/2 cup lettuce juice
> One teaspoon lemon juice

Stir vigorously to blend all ingredients and drink daily. This Raw Juice Heart Tranquilizer has substances including Vitamins A, C, E, and minerals that help promote a feeling of relaxation that is highly beneficial to the heart.

How RAW JUICE HEART TRANQUILIZER HELPED JEFF'S "AGING" HEART. In a reported case, Jeff M. suffered a coronary occlusion. He followed the prescribed course of all heart patients. No heavy lifting, lose weight, lower blood pressure, etc. His problem was high blood pressure and hypertension. His condition declined.

Has Chest Pains. In June, Jeff M. was at the peak of his angina pain. He was taking 20 nitroglycerine tablets daily. As a man with a wife and two small children to support, he became alarmed.

Seeks Natural Medical Help. He heard of a special clinic that used nutrition to promote health. Jeff M. had already been to two heart specialists and concluded that one more examination would not make his condition any worse, and might improve it. He made an appointment with the physician.

Given Raw Juice Heart Tranquilizer. When examined by the physician, he was given a complete physical and electrocardiogram. The diagnosis was the same as with the other two specialists—*a lack of oxygen in the left ventricle.* He was put on a special program using Vitamin E in combination with the above-mentioned vegetable and fruit juices. He was told to continue taking nitroglycerine tablets daily.

Increases Raw Juice Heart Tranquilizer. After a month, Jeff M. still had angina pain upon the least bit of exertion. His doctor told him to add more wheat germ oil to the raw juice drink to boost its potency.

Freedom From Chest Pain. Weeks went by and Jeff M. was still unrelieved. He was about to throw in the towel, accept defeat, and admit he was "taken for a ride." Then one day he awoke to a wonderful feeling. He was free of angina pain! His physician helped him decrease his intake of nitroglycerine tablets. His blood pressure dropped down to 120/80 and remained there. He continues with his nitroglycerine tablet treatment under doctor's orders, but found that his Raw Juice Heart Tranquilizer has eased his heart pain so much that he regards it as his all-natural relaxant. Jeff M. is now happy, healthy, and youthful.

BENEFITS OF RAW JUICE HEART TRANQUILIZER. In the preceding case, we note that Jeff's heart disorder was traced to a lack of oxygen in the left ventricle. It appears that the nutrients in the Raw Juice Heart Tranquilizer worked to provide the necessary oxygen and this created a wondrous feeling of a "young heart." The nutrients promoted an oxygenating action that helped distribute blood to all the vital body extremities.

RAW JUICES AND YOUTHFUL CELLULAR OXYGEN FOR THE HEART. Raw juices from fruits, vegetables and seeds promote a youthful cellular oxygen action for the heart. As a maintenance factor, the nutrients have a reduction-oxidation benefit that participates directly in the cellular exchanges of the body, possibly in the end stages of the metabolism of carbohydrates. The meaning of this is clear: reduction-oxidation, the physiological benefit of seed oils, is the inhibiting or reduction of the tendency of oxygen to combine with other substances and create stoppages. Raw juices are like air conditioning units to the body to maintain an even, calm and tranquil breath of life for the heart.

Look to seed and plant juices to help put youth into your heart and provide a soothing, healthful relaxation to nervous flutters. Let Nature enable you to drink your way to a young heart and a youthful life!

HIGHLIGHTS:

1. Seed juice is a rich source of the vitamin that reportedly helps promote heart rejuvenation. Wheat germ oil is a potent source of many other helpful nutrients.

2. The Heart Health Juice reportedly gave Bernice E. a new "heart-lease" on life.

3. Four "heart healing" benefits are provided by the Heart Health Juice.

4. A Raw Juice Heart Cocktail gives "second" life. Jack M. found new life and youth.

5. Grace J. feels young at 57, bouncing back from heart distress with the use of a corrective program and a Heart-Youth Tonic.

6. The Raw Juice Heart Tranquilizer gave Jeff M. a feeling of youth.

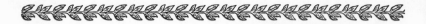

Chapter 12

How to Use Healthful Liquids

to Recharge Your Kidney-Liver

Power for Youthfulness

A prime source of "Young Again" vitality is to be found in the fresh live juices of fruits and vegetables that help invigorate the power of the kidney-liver combination. These two body organs are known for acting as filters, to help siphon off the age-causing toxic wastes and corrosive-acting remnants of metabolism. To help correct the problems of so-called "aging" fatigue and weakness, the kidneys and liver need to be properly nourished with emphasis upon two vital minerals—potassium and sodium. These two "Young Again" minerals are found in the live juices of plant foods. They serve to promote a good feeling through the regeneration of the kidneys and liver and thereby promote the look and feel of youth

HOW CERTAIN JUICES HELP REGENERATE
THE KIDNEYS

Live raw juices in plant foods help to nourish and re-generate the kidneys and help provide a feeling of youthful cleanliness. In particular, potassium (a mineral) has been seen to exert this beneficial youthfulness through kidney washing.

How Lester T. Used Live Juices to Improve Youthfulness.
Lester T. woke up feeling weak, fatigued. In his work as a stockroom supervisor, he had to lift comparatively heavy cartons which he had always done with ease. But one day, his muscles seemed to be working against him. Ordinary shipping chores became enormous tasks and drained him of what appeared to be every ounce of energy. Lester T. thought it would go away. The "weak feeling" did pass away. But it returned again and this time he had that awful feeling of being dragged down, sapped out of his strength. Now, he felt that he was getting old. When he dropped several cartons and broke expensive merchandise, his superior sent him for a physical examination.

Chronic Fatigue Traced to Internal Malnutrition. His prob-lem was chronic fatigue traced to internal under-nourishment and lack of sufficient kidney power. In an effort to avoid drugs (Lester always developed side effects from the slightest medication), he was given the following Internal Recharger Cocktail:

> 1/2 cup prune juice
> 1/2 cup orange juice
> 1/8 cup grapefruit juice

All the ingredients were to be thoroughly mixed together. Lester was to drink one Internal Recharger Cocktail about thirty minutes after each of his three daily meals. This Cocktail was a powerhouse of potassium to help wash and cleanse his internal organs, especially the kidneys. Here are the benefits:

Cleanses Kidney Filters. Potassium in the above live plant juices works to cleanse the kidney's filters. Many quarts of fluid pass through these filters daily and the potassium has a cleansing benefit similar to an antiseptic. Live fluid juices containing potassium promote this benefit.

Improves Circulation. Nutrients in the Internal Recharger Cocktail help invigorate the circulatory system to promote blood purification that could be sent streaming to all body parts and improve natural vitality.

Stimulates Metabolism. Potassium action through the kidneys works to stimulate the filters to strain waste products out of the blood, dissolve them in water and excrete them in wastes. Potassium then would take up valuable nutrients from digested food and work with enzymes to send them to all vital body parts where they would promote a youthful regeneration of body tissues and their functioning.

Maintains Healthful Water Balance. Nutrients in the Internal Recharger Cocktail help produce a natural water balance. A sluggish kidney loses its ability to regulate total body salt and water. Minerals help produce a natural balance and act as a healthful diuretic to stimulate kidney action.

LESTER T. ENJOYS A YOUTHFUL COMEBACK. In addition to the Internal Recharger Cocktail, Lester T. had to adjust his living program to include ample rest, recreation, and reduction of tensions; he found it difficult to eliminate artificial non-foods such as bleached flour products, pre-cooked meals, and large amounts of acid forming coffee. But when he was able to reduce his unnatural food intake and substitute with wholesome, natural foods, he enjoyed more of a youthful comeback. He had to use more fresh live juices rich in minerals and enzymes to stimulate a sluggish kidney-liver combination. Once this was accomplished, he could enjoy a youthful comeback. Packages no longer seemed heavy. Work was a joy. Nature had made all the difference! He drinks three glasses daily of the Internal Recharger Cocktail and finds himself in satisfying youthful health and able to cope with the physical demands of his job with ease.

HOW A POTASSIUM PUNCH HELPS KEEP
YOU FEELING YOUNGER

As a mineral found in live food juices, potassium has been seen to help keep you feeling and looking younger through healthy and normal kidney-liver functioning. True, it is good to be alive—but it is much better to feel youthful to enjoy being alive! Many folks find themselves growing weaker, seeing nothing more than years of dreary existence ahead of them. Many lament that it is little use to be alive when you are too tired to appreciate it. The truth is that many people grow potassium-deficient through insufficient live food juice intake with the passing of years, and so in weakening their kidney-liver power generators, they weaken themselves all over.

WHAT A POTASSIUM PUNCH CAN DO FOR YOU. When this mineral is squeezed out from living fruits and vegetables, and taken in the form of a Potassium Punch, the benefits are youthfully inspiring. Here are some known benefits of the Potassium Punch (recipe to follow in a few more paragraphs) as they can apply to you:

1. *Peps Up Youthful Muscularity.* Through its assimilation via the kidney-liver duo, the Potassium Punch strengthens the tissues and cells of the muscular system to promote youthful vitality. The sparse diet in weight control of many people results in a depletion of their potassium intake and a subsequent loss of normal muscular health results.

2. *Promotes Youthful Nerve Power.* The Potassium Punch nelps retain essential body fluids and metabolizes protein efficiently to help feed the nervous system sufficiently. Potassium ions are needed to balance sodium ions in relation to nerve conduction and muscular activity. This delicate but all-essential balance promotes a youthful nervous system through the Potassium Punch nutrients.

3. *Rejuvenates Strength.* There is a distinct relationship between youthful strength and nutrients in the Potassium Punch. In reported tests, doctors employed a right hand pressure grip called a dynamometer. This measured strength

among the elderly. Doctors took the average of three readings per person and compared them to normal values. They found that potassium becomes a powerhouse of strength-increasing action when taken in live food juices. The doctors reported that it is recognized scientifically "that administration of an adequate amount of potassium to depleted people restores strength significantly." All this in a natural live food juice!

4. *Regulates Youthful Metabolism.* The Potassium Punch sends living nutrients that are closely linked to the health of muscles, nerves and the metabolism process. Your blood pressure, your glands and hormones, depend to a large extent upon a sufficient amount of potassium in your body. The Potassium Punch is sent streaming through your kidney-liver duo, washing through, promoting a youthful metabolism for a more youthful body and appearance.

5. *Gives a Look and Feel Young Again Benefit.* A doctor reported that he treated a number of people over the age of 65. He found they were deficient in the ingredients found in the Potassium Punch. They were apathetic, underweight, listless, and depressed. Many of these symptoms seemed to be relieved when the kidney-liver function was revitalized through nutritional help and through the minerals found in the Potassium Punch.

How to Make Your Own Potassium Punch. You mix equal portions of any of the following live foods which are powerhouses of potassium: prunes, oranges, tangerines, grapefruits, figs, raisins, apricots, and cantaloupe. You may drink these raw juices in combination or singly. Just 1 glass will provide you with over 500 milligrams of this youthful mineral. It is beneficial to drink one glass in the morning, one at noontime and one in the evening.

HOW THE POTASSIUM PUNCH "REMADE" GRACE T.

As a piano teacner, Grace T. hardly had the time to prepare her own meals. She would usually "whip up something" with prepared mixes, packaged items, or pre-cooked foods in cartons. At age 46, she looked much older. She never thought it could be due to improper diet. She just thought she was working too hard in giving piano lessons almost seven days a week, working into the late hours of the night.

Feels Herself Getting Weaker. She began to grow weaker. Grace T. would be unable to finish the day with as much vitality as before. She took to drinking lots of black coffee but this only worsened the problem since caffeine provides a spurt of energy to be followed by a severe letdown. She soon was so weak, she could not even give morning piano lessons.

Tired Jaw Muscles Lead to Live Food Juices. Unable to chew properly, Grace T. had to cut down on her prepared foods and take to lots of natural juices. This proved to be a blessing in disguise. Her strength rallied. Grace T. found that live food juices prepared in her home juice extractor promoted a remarkable look and feel of youth. She prepared her own special *Second Youth Elixir:* Mix one-half cup apricot juice with one-half cup grapefruit juice. Add one tablespoon dark honey to ease the tart taste. Drink first thing in the morning.

BENEFITS: The Second Youth Elixir was a dynamic source of potassium that went directly to the kidney-liver duo and promoted a youthful function. Here is what happened in the system: the potassium in the Second Youth Elixir helped maintain normal osmotic pressure of the body fluids in the kidney-liver organs. The proper level of potassium *inside* the kidney-liver cells helped nourish the blood cells and muscles; also, the potassium worked to keep the proper level of potassium *outside* the kidney-liver cells, where it belongs, in the interstitial fluids such as blood serum and plasms. In Grace T.'s condition, sodium took over the kidney-liver cells, impaired filtering, leading to a health decline.

Second Youth Elixir Caused Rejuvenation. The potassium in this Second Youth Elixir was sent streaming to the red blood cells which effectively carried carbon dioxide through the blood to the lungs, where it was expelled in exchange for oxygen. Simultaneously, the potassium helped to maintain a slight alkalinity of the blood, a naturally nealthful condition.

The minerals and potassium in the Second Youth Elixir then acted as a *natural* diuretic by *stimulating the excretion of water by the kidneys, ridding the body of toxic age-causing waste materials.* This is its "magic" youth power.

Acts Upon Enzymes. Nutrients in the Second Youth Elixir activate certain enzymes needed for carbohydrate metabolism. Potassium is such an activator, sparking a healthful carbohydrate metabolism through the kidney-liver duo and creating an overall youthful feeling.

Processed Foods: Clues to Grace's Premature Aging. When the body is denied sufficient potassium, there is a feeling of weakness, neuromuscular functions become impaired, reflexes are poor, mental confusion takes place, and muscles turn soft and sag. Grace T. had these symptoms because the processed foods she ate were depleted and "robbed" of valuable minerals and also low in potassium. Food preservatives, additives, bleaches, and chemicalization all tend to deplete and destroy potassium supply. Grace T. learned that the artificial seasoning in such bleached foods created this potassium-depletion. By selecting natural foods and by taking a Second Youth Elixir regularly, she helped create a healthful balance. She became energetic once again. We hope she will continue to use Nature's live food juices to enjoy a young-again life.

HOW A LIVER-CLEANSING PROGRAM PROMOTES "LOOK ALIVE" FEELING

The liver is the largest organ in the body. Located on the right side of the abdomen, a little beneath the waist line, the liver must always be kept cleansed to perform its "look alive" function at top efficiency. A thoroughly cleansed liver will do the following to promote the look and feel of youth:

1. It changes (metabolizes) carbohydrates into glycogen which it then stores and releases to the body to provide youthful energy when needed.

2. A cleansed liver breaks down fats so they may be burned or oxidized in the cells.

3. A cleansed liver passes bile off into the excretory system; this is the residue left from the breakdown of red blood cells. Good health requires normal release of bile.

4. A healthy liver acts as a storage site for iron and fibrogen, two blood substances that promote healing.

5. A youthful liver stores Vitamin D, needed to promote strong bones and muscles.

6. A healthy liver is a storage depot for the blood-forming factor, producing the substances from which healthy young blood is made.

7. A healthy liver keeps you young by absorbing from the digestive tract those poisons which might otherwise be fatal or rob one of youthfulness.

THREE-DAY LIQUID LIVER REJUVENATION PROGRAM. Here is a fasting program designed to help cleanse the liver to promote the preceding seven benefits that create a "look alive" feeling:

First Day: $1/8$ glass raw beet (and greens) juice. Sip slowly. Mix together two quarts water plus two cups fresh lemon juice. Add two tablespoons raw honey. Drink whenever you desire throughout the first day.

Second Day: $1/4$ glass raw beet (and greens) juice. Sip slowly. Drink the lemon water as described above.

Third Day: One glass raw beet (and greens) juice. Sip slowly. Drink the lemon water as described above.

AFTER THE 3-DAY FAST: Begin solid foods by taking any raw grated vegetable and any raw juice in any desired amount. Gradually, take ground nuts or seeds with raw fruit and vegetable juices. On the seventh day, eat lightly of a mild protein food such as natural cheese, coddled eggs, sprouts of any kind, nut or seed milk, or steamed vegetables. Afterwards, return to a normal and natural eating program.

BENEFITS OF THE "THREE-DAY LIQUID LIVER REJUVENATION PROGRAM." Roy T. had found himself looking pale and wan. In addition, he developed such indigestion that whatever he ate would "come back" on him. He endured severe colitis that further depleted his health.

Roy T. ate for *taste* rather than *health*. He was somewhat "addicted" to bleached foods, prepared and processed dishes and this depleted his precious mineral content. His liver suffered. So did his health!

He underwent this special three day fast, helped promote a vigorous liver that was able to metabolize carbohydrates into energy producing glycogen, cleanse the bile from the body, improve Vitamin D storage and eventual assimilation, and rid the body of toxic age-causing wastes. These benefits through the minerals in the beets and other live foods helped improve his liver—and his health.

However, Roy T. could not give up his processed, overly seasoned non-foods and his health declined to the point where malfunctioning kidney-liver upset led to hospitalization. This might have been averted through live food juices!

YOGA SECRET OF LIVER MASSAGE. At a leading health farm, yoga lessons include this simple but surprisingly effective Liver Massaging Exercise:

Lie on the floor, or on a slant board, with head down. Pull knees up to chest. Hug with your arms. Return feet out straight and hands over head. Repeat five times. Repeat the Liver Massaging Exercise three times daily. It helps release the stored up sluggish wastes and with the use of potassium through live food juices, promotes a remarkably soothing cleansing of this vital organ.

HOW A POTASSIUM POTION PROMOTED HEALTHFUL BLOOD PRESSURE

Roger T. felt a decline in his appetite. He should have known that this is Nature's warning signal that a malfunctioning kidney-liver duo means a loss of minerals. Roger T. then showed nervous disorders but most serious of all, a high blood pressure.

Mystery of High Blood Pressure. It is reported that doctors could not reduce Roger T.'s blood pressure with drugs. They further learned that Roger T. had a potassium deficiency. Frequently, tension accelerates potassium loss and Roger T.

was very tense. This set up a chain reaction in the glands in which the adrenal produces hormones that deplete the potassium supply. Roger T. grew very nervous until doctors found that it was partially traced to his potassium deficiency.

POTASSIUM TONIC TURNS THE TIDE. A high potassium live juice was prepared of an equal portion of apricots, cantaloupe, and oranges. This sent a powerhouse of potassium to the kidney-liver filters and helped to promote better health. *But* his high blood pressure still did not come down to normal. Roger T.'s diet was carefully checked: the culprit was *licorice!* This non-food has ammonium glycyrrhizate which causes sodium retention, potassium diuresis, and shoots up the blood pressure. By eliminating the licorice candy, giving Roger the Potassium Tonic, his blood pressure reportedly came down to normal.

Furthermore, kidney-liver health and potassium nourishment eased and eliminated his so-called paralysis or stiffness; his muscles became charged with strength. He was on the way to youthful recovery. Let us hope he takes several glasses of the Potassium Tonic daily.

HOW RAW JUICES PROMOTE HEART HEALTH. The Potassium Tonic also promotes heart health, your body's most active muscle. In the heart, potassium deficiency leads to muscle degeneration, necrosis, connective tissue degeneration, and cellular edema, as in other tissue cells. Raw juices and the Potassium Tonic benefit the heart by removing fluids from the body. But the Potassium Tonic is reportedly *more* beneficial than some diuretics because the latter cause a mineral depletion. A Potassium Tonic helps maintain a normal level in the heart muscle.

LOOK TO NATURE. Raw juices are healthful sources of potassium in contrast to the pharmaceutical preparations which often have an irritating effect on the kidney-liver-intestinal network. Pharmaceutical preparations may create excessive levels of potassium that upset the delicate kidney-liver-intestinal balance. So—look to Nature for your potassium

For the "Young Again" vitality, renourish your kidney-liver combination through proper minerals found in live raw juices. This helps recharge your "youth power" to promote a vibrant mind and body. It's all there—in Nature, for the drinking!

IMPORTANT BENEFITS:

1. Lester T. used a simple all-natural Internal Recharger Cocktail to help wash his kidney-liver duo and promote the look and feel of youth.
2. A Potassium Punch offers five "young again" benefits.
3. The Second Youth Elixir promoted Grace T.'s rejuvenation.
4. A simple "liver-cleansing" program promotes a "look alive" feeling.
5. Obtain 7 distinct benefits for a healthy liver via the Three Day Liver Rejuvenation program. It's easy!
6. A Potassium Potion reportedly normalized Roger T.'s blood pressure and rescued him from premature aging.
7. A healthy kidney-liver-intestine-heart network is possible through minerals, enzymes and nutrients found in live raw juices.

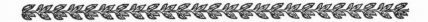

Chapter 13

The Raw Juice Program to Help

Promote "Happy Glands" for

a Youthful Personality

As an automobile salesman, Dennis C. displayed such an irascible temperament that prospective customers would walk out of the showroom in anger. Dennis C. had not always been so jumpy, short-tempered, or sarcastic. At one time, he had been a smooth talker, using a glib line that would sell many cars to happy customers. But he gradually developed a jittery personality that led to snappy remarks and an unpleasant disposition. This negative personality cost him many commission dollars and lost his firm a lot of customers.

Raw Juice Program Corrects "Angry" Glands. When Dennis C. underwent a routine health examination, it was noted that his blood sugar was extremely low. His gland-hormonal network required improvement. He was placed on a special high-protein, low-sugar raw juice program. This helped promote a gradual tranquilization of his hormonal rhythm; it eased his low blood sugar condition of *hypoglycemia* and helped correct his problem of "angry" glands.

Protein Juice: Dennis C. was told to drink three cups daily of this special Protein Juice:

> 1/4 cup tomato juice
> 4 tablespoons desiccated liver powder
> 2 tablespoons lemon juice
> 1/4 cup carrot juice

Mix thoroughly together and drink slowly. The benefit here is that minerals in the tomato and carrot juices promote a steady absorption of the amino acids in the desiccated liver powder. (This is sold at most health food stores. It is a powder made of whole liver, with the connective tissue, bone, and fat removed.) In harmony, the symphony of these nutrients helped stimulate sluggish glands and provided a *gradual* assimilation of food for the hormones.

Soon Dennis C. felt happy, developed a winning personality, and was able to sell many more cars. A raw juice program provided protein food to his hormonal network and promoted this look and feel of a "young personality." His temperament was optimistically cheerful, thanks to correction of low blood sugar through raw juices.

HOW PROTEIN JUICES HELP REJUVENATE "AGED" GLANDS

The problem faced by Dennis C. is one that is responsible for many so-called "aging" disorders involving the problem of so-called senility, namely, irascible, grouchy, gloomy, and depressive emotional conditions that are erroneously attributed to "getting old." Doctors report that protein juices are able to stabilize the gland-hormonal system through correction of blood sugar and thereby improve and rejuvenate the entire network to promote a "happy" personality that is reflective of carefree, youthful personalities.

Protein Juice: Food for Young Glands. A supply of bubbling amino acids from assimilated protein juices becomes food for the glands to promote "young hormones" and a "young personality." These amino acids enter into the ductless glands (so called because their secretions or hormones do not pass through tubes or ducts, but pour out directly into the bloodstream) and create a youthful treasure of benefits. The amino acids from protein juices influence the seven important glands, from the head downward: the pituitary, thyroid, parathyroids, thymus, adrenals, pancreas, and gonads.

The amino acids from seed juices influence the glands to create growth, development, tissue regeneration, muscular tone, and resistance to fatigue. These same amino acids influence the amount of hormones produced and their regulation and function in the body. The protein juices send amino acids to influence emotions as well as physical responses. A deficiency of sufficient protein juices may cause the glands to produce too many or too few hormones and this may create emotional disorders that have been classified as "schizophrenic" in more severe situations. Seed juices may well hold the clue to creating a youthful personality.

How Louise T. Used a Protein Juice to Correct Her Aging Gland-Personality. Louise T. found housework to be more laborious as time went on. Although she was in her late 30's, she felt she was in her late 60's. A small bundle of laundry was a dead weight. The few dishes in the sink appeared mountainous. Little noises were sonic booms to her. She lost her temper upon the slightest provocation; she was nervous, snappy, and irritable. Her family noticed this personality derangement and thought it was the onset of premature aging. Louise T. developed such intense recurring spells of exhaustion, weakness, and depression that she had to go to the doctor.

Actually, Louise T. feared she had diabetes since she knew it was a genetic disorder and "runs in the family." Both of her parents had diabetes. Now, was she falling victim to this ailment?

This fear led to the doctor visit. He made a complete examination and said that she did *not* have any diabetic problem. However, her nervous-emotional derangement was due to a hormonal imbalance and low blood sugar.

Blood Sugar Health. The doctor explained that normal blood sugar is 80 milligrams to 100 milligrams per 100 cubic centimeters of blood, under a doctor's test. But if the diet is deficient in protein, among other nutrients, the blood sugar curve shoots upward and then plummets downward again.

Value of Blood Sugar. The doctor explained that the body converts starchy foods into *glucose* which is carried by the blood to every body cell for heat and energy. In usual circumstances, part of the glucose is immediately metabolized. The rest is stored in the liver and in muscle tissue to be used between meals to promote glandular energy and personality youth. This helps maintain a proper level of blood glucose.

Imbalance Causes Personality "Aging." A protein-deficient bloodstream means that there is an imbalance of glucose. With a shortage of glucose in the blood, there is a form of *cell starvation* that causes low blood sugar or hypoglycemia. This creates "aging glands" and a personality wrecking attitude that is self-destructive. The key to stabilization of a "happy glandular" condition is to obtain sufficient amino acids through protein juices and feed a regular supply of glucose into the hormonal network.

Louise T.'s Special Protein Juice for Happy Glands. Louise T. was told to mix 1/2 cup soybean powder together with 1 1/2 cups water. Blend at high speed for 3 to 4 minutes. Strain through a cheese cloth. Drink this Protein Juice, freshly made, three times daily.

Benefits: About one cup of this Protein Juice sends 75 grams of nutrients streaming into the digestive system to become assimilated into the bloodstream and to feed the hormonal network with a rich supply of amino acids. These amino acids then help maintain a healthful and youthful supply of glucose in the system, to promote a cheerful personality and "happy glands." Louise T. was told to eliminate concentrated sugar foods which interfered with a steady and tranquil amino acid metabolism. It was this corrective program with three daily cups of the Protein Juice that helped transform Louise T. into a "youthful" woman and the cheerful personality of one who had "happy glands." Protein had helped effect this look and feel of youth!

How a Sugar-Free Program Made Richard C. Feel Young Again. Richard C. as a printer and sometime proofreader, found his tedious work suffering from recurring mistakes. Richard C. was troubled with headaches, stomach spasms, drowsiness and blurring of the senses. Proof sheets looked blurred; lines were confused; errors were not caught; and customers complained. Richard C. was in threat of losing his job to a younger man.

Richard C. Was A Sugar-holic. His problem was an excessive amount of sugar via the printing plant's readily available soda vending machine as well as the "snack bar" with packaged, processed candy, cake and confection non-foods. Richard C. consumed so much of this foodless snack supply that he became a "sugar-holic." The problem here is that the *rapidly absorbed carbohydrates* played havoc with his blood sugar, yanking the levels upward and then plummeting downward. Richard's glands had to metabolize the speedy carbohydrates in this somewhat vicious up-and-down process and this caused his emotional distress.

How Emotional Youth Reacts to Unhappy Glands. An excess of non-food sugar put more work on the endocrine glands such as the pituitary, thyroid, and adrenals; they were forced to manufacture more hormones to elevate blood sugar. Then, the speedily metabolized carbohydrate caused a drop in blood sugar and this upset Richard's hormonal level. His emotional vitality was likewise influenced by the "unhappy gland" condition and his mental health declined. He was tired, sleepy, disorganized, easily upset, grouchy, and temperamental. He did not know it was caused by the consumption of so much sugar.

How Seed Milks Promote Youthful Gland Health. A natural health nutritionist suggested he prepare the following:

Seed Milk for Young Glands

$^1/_2$ cup sesame seeds (available at health stores)

$1^1/_2$ cups water

Blend at high speed for 4 minutes. Strain through cheesecloth. Add dark organic honey to taste. Drink slowly.

Benefit: The sesame seed milk is rich in easily assimilated amino acids and natural carbohydrates. The honey has a "stabilizer" in its minerals to help promote a gradual absorption of the amino acids to promote young gland health.

Eliminate Sugar Foods. Richard C. had to eliminate all non-foods containing sugar. No more candy, cake, snacks, or soda pop drinks. It took several weeks for his glands to recuperate and Richard C. no longer felt dizzy, blurred, nervous, or old. He had young glands, thanks to the Seed Milk for Young Glands that he drank three times daily. Now he could hold onto his job. He felt younger than young!

GROWS YOUNGER WITH "HAPPY HORMONE ELIXIR." In one reported case, Ida C., at age 50, came to her doctor with health problems. She had severe headaches in the back of her head and distressful sinusitis. Nightly, she had to get up a few times to make "bathroom trips." She suffered from chronic constipation.

Ida C. had an insatiable craving for candy. She ate as much as two pounds a week! She awakened exhausted and remained exhausted all day long. She also suffered from mental depression.

HAPPY HORMONE ELIXIR. A program called for the elimination of sugar and white flour to help correct her glandular distress. Ida C. benefitted from this special:

Happy Hormone Elixir

1 cup cashew nut powder (ground on a mill)

2 tablespoons rice polish (found at health stores)

2 cups water

Put in blender and whir 4 to 5 minutes. Add one tablespoon honey to taste

Benefits: A powerhouse of amino acids and minerals combine to nourish the hormonal system and provide a tranquil blood sugar.

Ida C. was reported as recovering in just two weeks. She was free from sensitivity to extreme temperature of food. She had just one headache. Her sinus condition improved. She slept well throughout the night. She awakened with youthful energy. Her husband said she was more cheerful and youthful, thanks to happy hormones! The only remaining problem is that she still had a craving for sweets. If this could be eased, then she would feel young again. Ida C. has now helped control her urge for sweets, followed the sugar-free and white flour-free program, and with the help of amino acids, actually drank her way to happy hormones.

WHY SEED JUICES HELP BUILD HAPPY GLANDS. Seeds are rich in amino acids as well as vitamins and minerals. The benefit here is that a high-protein and low-starch program promotes a youthful glandular condition. Protein and fats are assimilated much more slowly than carbohydrates (starches and sugars) and so do not produce a rush of sugar. Slow burning, they are long-lasting fuels to help maintain a delightful personality through happy glands. Seed juices are prime sources of this high-protein and low-starch program.

Drink Seed Milks Daily: To promote the look and feel of young glands, drink home-made seed milks daily. At health stores, you will find sunflower seeds, squash and pumpkin seeds, sesame seeds, as well as soybeans which are dynamic sources of gland-needing amino acids. Mix one-half cup of seed powder with water and drink slowly. (Use a moderate amount of honey, which is a concentrated source of carbohydrates yet has beneficial hormone-needing minerals.)

Eliminate coffee, cola and other sweet soft drinks, nonfoods such as sugary candy, cakes, pastries, confections, and pies. Coffee and cola drinks contain caffeine which causes an unpleasant up-and-down blood sugar yank that leads to emotional-personality derangement. Substitute wholesome seed milks, soybean juices, fresh vegetable juices, coffee substitutes, or herbal teas. For snacks, use sunflower seeds, nuts, or carob candy in moderation (sold at health stores).

Help your hormones enjoy a happy disposition through raw seed juices. Hormones are the sparkplugs of a young feeling. Nourish them with natural foods and live raw juices. With seed juices you can be of good cheer!

IN REVIEW:

1. Dennis C. corrected his "angry" glands and developed a youthfully winning personality with a special raw juice program.

2. The Protein Juice made of several ingredients helped feed the hormonal system to promote a youthful personality.

3. A special Protein Juice for Happy Glands put Louise T. back on the road to youth.

4. A sugar-free program plus Seed Milk for Young Glands made Richard C. feel younger-than-young.

5. The Happy Hormone Elixir promoted a feeling of new youth for Ida C.

6. Seed juices and seed milks help build happy glands.

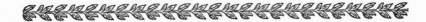

Chapter 14

The 5-Step Liquid Food Program

that Helps Banish Headaches

A mind that is youthfully alert and free from head-aches is one that can do miracles of creativity. Nature fully intended the human mind to enjoy the benefits of the look and feel of youth, just as the human body enjoys the invigoration of healthful living. Liquid foods have been known to promote a form of "emotional rejuvenation" that helps relax-relieve tensions and abolish the necessity of aspirin chemicalization.

HOW AN ASPIRIN-FREE PROGRAM REBUILT STEVE'S EMOTIONAL YOUTH

As high-pressure sales manager, Steve T. was constantly beset with headaches, pains in the back of his neck, pounding heart, sweaty palms, and nervous disorders. His work sched-ule was so heavy with so many sales meetings and calls that he was on the go from early morning to late in the evening. This particular overload of work and constant tension resulted in his recurring headaches.

Steve T. had to keep up with competing youngsters so he kept taking an assortment of aspirins and so-called pain-killers. He hoped these would deaden the pain, relieve the tensions and give him the emotional energy and youth he needed to continue his sales job. He also had worries that younger salesmen with more emotional health and strength would take away some of his business. He relied upon aspirins to the degree that he took about six per day. He also took many pain killers, tension-easers, and other chemicals that promised him relief. Then he noticed a decline in mental vigor.

Aspirins Slowed Down Thyroid Gland. His excessive aspirin medication caused his thyroid gland to become slowed down. Steve T. felt weak, disinterested, frequently dizzy, even unable to add up a small column of figures. His thoughts became sluggish. At times, he gave the impression of being senile and he was all of 45! He was examined by a company doctor and told that salicylates (medical name for aspirins and pain killers) interfered with the production of a hormone which stimulates the thyroid into youthful activity. Salicylates slow down the action of the thyroid gland. When the hormone thyroxin is diminished, it becomes underactive, and there is a form of "aging" that causes emotional and physical decline. *Aspirins were making him old before his time!*

Turns to Liquid Foods for Freedom from Headaches. He was told to make a simple all-natural liquid food that would help relax his nervous system and promote resistance to tension. Steve T. had to give up his aspirins, too. Here is the beverage he made:

Nature's Tension-Eze Tonic
4 tablespoons brewer's yeast flakes
1 tablespoon fenugreek herb seeds
2 tablespoons dark organic honey

Heat two cups of water. When bubbly hot, add the brewer's yeast flakes, the fenugreek herb seeds, and stir vigorously.

Let them steep about ten minutes. Pour off through a strainer into a cup. Add the honey. Drink slowly.

How Nature's Tension-Eze Tonic Promotes Headache Relief. The brewer's yeast flakes are a prime source of the B-complex vitamins which are needed to nourish and strengthen the nervous system. The fenugreek herb seeds (sold at all health food stores) contain all-natural ingredients needed to give a tranquil and relaxed emotional system. The honey is a good source of minerals that send forth a "smoothing balm" upon the vascular nervous system and help ease the tight constriction that causes nervous tension headaches.

It is this 3-step benefit, working in a marvelous "time release" program (it works slowly, one step at a time) that helps bring about a general relaxation of the nervous system to promote a youthful well-being.

Steve T. Now Looks and Thinks Young. By eliminating aspirins, cutting down his work load, and taking Nature's Tension-Eze Tonic, Steve T. found his thoughts more youthful and energetic. He could look and think young again, much better than his younger competitors! His headache problem may be corrected if he will learn to ease up on his work schedule and follow the natural laws of healthful living. Let us hope he continues taking two cups of Nature's Tension-Eze Tonic daily—for his head's sake!

THE 5-STEP LIQUID FOOD PROGRAM THAT HELPS BANISH HEADACHES

Nature's liquid foods contain ingredients that help you "think young" and strengthen resistance against tension-causing headaches. The secret here is that in liquid form, these ingredients go speedily to work, directly to the *cause* of the distress, thereby easing the symptoms. Liquids are assimilated much faster than solids, the ingredients are much more speedily metabolized by a nerve-health system craving relief. Here is a special 5-Step Liquid Food Program to help banish headaches and promote a "think young" exhilaration:

1—"FOREVER YOUNG SEED JUICE"

Investigators have found that a simple seed juice, namely wheat germ oil, has been able to promote a "forever young" emotional health.

How to Make Forever Young Seed Juice: Mix six table-spoons of wheat germ oil in one glass of fresh carrot juice. Add several sprinkles of lemon juice for a tangy flavor. Stir vigorously. Drink one glass in the morning, another glass at noon, and a final glass in the evening.

Benefits: This particular Forever Young Seed Juice is a prime source of Vitamin C and Vitamin E. The benefit here is that Vitamin E preserves the oxygen in the blood for extended periods. This means smoother efficiency as blood is pumped through the blood vessels of the head which figure so promi-nently in headaches. Vitamin C works with Vitamin E to keep the blood vessels flexible, healthy, and less sensitive to painful disturbances. The Vitamin A also helps stabilize the action of the other nutrients to promote a *gradual* absorp-tion-assimilation to help build day-long and night-long relaxa-tion and freedom from the causes of headaches. In turn, the improved oxygenation helps refresh-aerate the nervous sys-tem to promote youthful mental exhilaration. The Forever Young Seed Juice promotes a young emotional health.

2—SALAD JUICE FOR "MIND FOOD"

Dorothy U. is a successful career woman in a big city. She competes with younger women and nearly always emerges as the successful one because she has such a "young outlook" and a vivid constructive imagination. At age 56, Dorothy U. is much sought after by many advertising agencies for her creative, forward looking ideas. She looks and thinks young. She has not taken any aspirins for more years than she cares to recall. She is able to refresh-rejuvenate-rebuild her thoughts and enjoy freedom from headaches because twice daily, she has Salad Juice for "Mind Food."

How to Make Salad Juice for "Mind Food": Whether dining out or dining in, Dorothy U. asks or prepares a small dish of freshly washed and scrubbed seasonal green leafy vegetables.

She then has two cups of simmering water prepared freshly. She soaks the vegetables in the water for just a few moments. This helps extract valuable vitamins and minerals. She then adds a little honey to the water and she drinks this unique Salad Juice. (She also eats the vegetables.)

Benefits: The coarse green leaves of raw vegetables are rich in vitamins, minerals, and enzymes. Just as juicing helps bring them out of their cellulose envelopes, so this "hot soak" for just a few moments helps bring out precious nutrients in a juice form that goes to work within moments after Dorothy U. has swallowed it. The nutrients help promote a nerve-vascular relaxation that enables a fresh oxygen-bearing bloodstream to reach the thought-creating centers of the brain. This helps give Dorothy the "mind food" that promotes the look and feel of a young mind! A simple and all-natural Salad Juice for "Mind Food" makes her younger than young!

3—"Think Young Toddy"

A time-tested folk healer is a simple but powerfully effective apple juice toddy. Many folks report that when a hot toddy is prepared and consumed several times a day, the ingredients are able to promote an overall youthful benefit. Many feel that headaches can be banished by corrective living and the use of a "Think Young Toddy"—to be taken instead of a chemical aspirin.

How to Make Your "Think Young Toddy": Prepare one or two glasses of fresh apple juice. Simmer in a kettle. Add one-half teaspoon cinnamon powder. Stir vigorously. Let cool and sip slowly.

Benefits: The warm apple juice is soothingly calm to the metabolism. It is also a prime source of Vitamin A that helps work together with calcium and phosphorus to promote a stabilized nerve strength. One particular benefit here is that the slight simmering provides a special "energetic-activation" of the minerals to help the body absorb iron so that the bloodstream is able to transport youth-bestowing oxygen to the arterial network. Furthermore, the cinnamon addition is a special benefit because this herbal spice contains plant extractives that stimulate the circulation to promote a refreshment of congested nervous pocket sites. This mutual benefit has made the "Think Young Toddy" a much desired liquid food to help relieve head pains and stimulate youthful energy. It's an old time folk healer that has been handed down throughout the generations. It helps the body stay young and think young longer.

4—BARLEY BREW FOR BETTER BRAIN POWER

Barley is a cereal popular in many parts of the world for bread-making. Barley is a time-tested folk healer known to the lake dwellers in ancient Switzerland. Here is an all-natural seed that is brimming in nerve-strengthening and brain-boosting B-complex vitamins. Barley can often provide a revitalization through all-natural carbohydrate metabolization that promotes remarkable thinking power.

How to Make Your Barley Brew for Better Brain Power: Add one tablespoon of organic unsprayed barley to two cups of piping hot water. Stir vigorously to dissolve as much as possible. Sip slowly. Eat the rest with a spoon.

Benefits: The concentrated food elements including B-complex and also some amino acids work together to help send a fresh stream of energy to the nerve network, helping to relax the constriction and thereby provide much needed nourishment to the processes concerned with mental youth. Many people will have two cups of Barley Brew at breakfast time to provide them with the foundation for a day of "think young" emotional health.

5—HAPPY WHEY TONIC

The magic ingredient in whey is the mineral calcium. Here is a dynamic mineral that is able to exert a magnetic action, drawing away excess fluids from the congested parts of the nervous system and promote a relieved-relaxed frame of "think young" mental health.

Whey is the remaining liquid taken from yogurt and milk. It is regarded the plasma part of milk—whole milk modified by a lactic acid culture, with curds and butterfat removed. Dried whey powder, when dehydrated without excess heat, reportedly contains twenty times the mineral content of liquid milk and fifty times as much lactose or milk sugar as yogurt or buttermilk. The mineral helps promote mental rejuvenation while the lactose promotes an internal cleansing that removes "cobwebs" and "frustrations" traced to vascular congestion. This unique benefit makes whey a miracle mind-booster. Whey powder is sold at almost all health food stores.

How to Make Your Happy Whey Tonic: Mix two tablespoons of whey powder in one cup of simmered water. Stir vigorously. Add mineral-rich dark organic honey to taste. Sip slowly.

Benefits: This particular Happy Whey Tonic was the answer to the headaches-tension-chronic mental fatigue of Vivian G. At a young 40, Vivian found each day growing longer and longer. She suffered from severe headaches that were like migraines. She had blurring of vision, occasional nausea, and a one-side-of-the-head "paralysis" feeling. She complained she often felt that half of her head was squeezed into a merciless tight vise. It would squeeze tighter and tighter as her tasks mounted up. Aspirins dulled some of the pain but caused such allergic reactions that she had to give them up.

Unable to drink milk because it gave her a "gagged" feeling, she turned to whey. She liked the taste of whey; but more than its liquid velvet smoothness, she liked the way it reduced the pounding of her headaches. She soon learned that whey could actually relax-rejuvenate her emotional state so she could have freedom from headaches.

The Happy Whey Tonic that Vivian G. used, was a prime source of carefully balanced calcium-phosphorus minerals as well as vitamins, that promoted these youth-giving benefits: These nutrients relaxed the swelling (dilation) of the arteries of the head which led to the pain-sensitive swollen blood vessels. Once this was done, the minerals then helped to create relaxing of the pulling (traction) that tension developed. The minerals cooled the inflamed arteries that were responsible for much pain. The next blessed benefit of the nutrients in the Happy Whey Tonic was the way they soothed and eased the swollen arteries and inflammation of the muscular-contractions in the neck, so often associated with headache distress and "too tired to think clearly" distress.

Vivian G. was able to enjoy freedom from the *causes* of her headache problem and with the use of minerals in the Happy Whey Tonic, was able to ease constriction of the tight blood vessels, relax the distension or swelling and soothe the pain of the engorged arterial walls of the upper extremities.

Vivian G. now feels young, thinks young, and looks young. True, the Happy Whey Tonic was not the only program used. Vivian G. had to obtain more sleep, reduce her reading and eyestrain, get away from noisy environments, and ease up on her work schedule. But with the use of Happy Whey Tonic, she fed herself relaxation from *within* while she promoted relaxation from *without*. This double-barrelled program helped banish her headaches and promote a stimulation of youthful thoughts.

REJUVENATE WITH NATURE. To look and feel young without headaches, observe the drugless laws of Nature. Ease up on excessive work; cut down on tension-causing situations. Enjoy your work, enjoy your home, enjoy your all-natural food. With the use of liquid foods, you can rejuvenate your insides. With the use of natural outside surroundings, you can rebuild your outsides. Together, you can help banish headaches and stimulate young thoughts with the 5-step liquid food program.

IN REVIEW:

1. How a headache-free program rebuilt Steve's youth without aspirin.
2. Nature's Tension-Eze Tonic helps strengthen nervous health and promote youthful happiness.
3. A special selection of five liquid foods, easily prepared in your own home, helps promote "forever young" emotional

health. A suggestion is to use all five tonics, dividing them up to be taken one a day. This helps promote a headache-free hope for emotional health.

4. Build youthfulness with the use of these all-natural liquid refreshers: Forever Young Seed Juice, Salad Juice for Mind Food, Think Young Toddy, Barley Brew for Better Brain Power, and Happy Whey Tonic. Rejuvenate your mind—with natural methods.

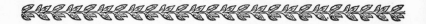

Chapter 15

Herb Tonics—Nature's Youth

Medicines to Replace Drugs

and Patent Medicines

THE ancients, in their quest for eternal youth, relied upon the magical and often mystical ingredients found in herbs. Many reportedly discovered herbal healers that could correct lifelong illnesses, ease so-called aging problems, and help rebuild the power of youth in body and mind. In the days before drugs and chemical patent medicines, herbs were Nature's youth medicines. These healing grasses were found to contain amazing youth restoratives that helped the body tap its own hidden sources of rejuvenation, to create a "young again" feeling. Herbs, as Nature's Youth Medicines are gradually being revived in our modern time in the hope for healing through drug-free potions. Herbs may be used by you to help promote your look and feel of youth—the Nature Way.

HOW HERB POTIONS PROMOTE NATURAL YOUTH

Herbs are prime sources of ingredients that reportedly will perform the following benefits to promote natural youth: *Anodyne* action to relieve pain; *aperient* action to promote a natural laxative benefit; *astringent* to cause healing; *antibilious* to act on bile and relieve bilious feeling; *antiemetic* to control nausea; *antilitic* to cleanse calculi from the urinary organs; *antiscorbutic* to relieve scurvy and rebuild young-again skin tissues; *anti-rheumatic* to relieve rheumatic-arthritic stiffness generally associated with older years; *antiseptic* to promote regeneration; *antispasmodic* to relieve spasms; *cathartic* to promote bowel movement without harsh chemical action; *cephalic* to oxygenate the mental processes; *cholagogue* to increase liquid flow and correct circulation; *condiment* to put flavor in food; *demulcent* to soothe and relieve inflammation; *deobstruent* to remove obstructions; *depurative* to purify the bloodstream; *detergent* to cleanse boils, wounds, cuts and lacerations; *diaphoretic* to produce normal and healthful perspiration and self-cleansing; *discutient* to dissolve and eliminate decaying tissues; *diuretic* to induce a natural flow of wastes; *emollient* to soften and soothe inflamed parts; *esculent* as a food; *exanthematous* as a folk remedy to heal the skin; *febrifuge* to abate and reduce fevers; *hepatic* to regenerate the liver and create youthful metabolism; *herpatic* to cleanse the skin and promote detoxification; *laxative* to promote natural bowel action; *lithontryptic* to dissolve and cast off waste substances in the system.

Maturating to promote expulsion of waste tissues and decaying, age-causing cells; *mucilaginous* to soothe inflamed parts; *nervine* to allay nervous excitement and control the nervous system; *opthalmicum* to promote youthful visual health; *pectoral* to relieve chest afflictions; *refrigerant* to cool the body; *resolvent* to dissolve and remove decaying wastes; *rubifacient* to increase circulation and promote a youthful glow; *sedative* to quiet upset nerves; *sialagogue* to increase mouth enzymes and help induce youthful digestion; *stomachic* to strengthen and give youthful tonus to the digestive organs; *styptic* to induce better healing of wounds; *sudorific* to produce needed perspiration and promote self-cleansing; *vermifuge* to expel worms.

The ancients recognized these and many more "young again" properties of Nature's healing grasses. If it is true that ancients lived for hundreds of years, perhaps herbs held the answer to their prolonged youth. Herbs are available today and should be used as part of the program to promote the look and feel of youth.

WHERE TO OBTAIN HERBS. Inquire at any local health food store. Look in the classified telephone directory under "herbs" and "herbal pharmacies." Many such stores have mail order services that are available for your convenience. Select fresh, organically grown herbs.

FOUR TYPES OF HERBS AND HOW TO USE THEM

Generally speaking, herbs are available in these four types, depending upon your personal preferences. Here is how to use herbs in these four types:

1. *Granulated or finely cut herbs*. Steep one heaping teaspoonful of the herbs in one cup of boiling water for twenty minutes. Strain. Take one cup an hour before each meal and one cup upon retiring. You may take more or less as the case requires. If too strong, use less herbs per cup.

2. *Roots and barks*. Simmer roots and barks for 30 minutes, or longer, in order to extract their healing ingredients. Do not boil hard. If the tea is too strong, add more water.

3. *Flowers and leaves*. Steep flowers and leaves in boiling water in a covered kettle for twenty minutes. Do not boil since this evaporates the aromatic properties.

4. *Powdered herbs*. Mix powdered herbs with either hot or cold water. Use one-half teaspoonful to one-fourth glass of water. Follow by drinking one glass water, either hot or cold. The herbs take effect quicker if taken in hot water.

FOR ADDED FLAVOR: Take a little honey in your herb tonic

to make it more palatable. Do *not* use any form of sugar. Do *not* prepare herbs or any food in aluminum cooking utensils—use stainless steel or pyrex-treated glass. Do *not* take drugs or patent medicines when taking Nature's own youth herbs since they do not work together. You may add a little fruit or vegetable juice to the herb tonic to increase its taste.

HOW FRANCES E. FOUND YOUTHFUL REGULARITY WITH HERBS

Frances E. was troubled with so-called "middle age" irregularity even though she was in her late 30's. She felt drained out by the vicious laxative habit. She fell victim to colitis because of the harsh action of chemical purgatives and laxatives. When her pharmacy was sold out on a much-advertised chemical laxative, she started looking for another pharmacy and found one that specialized in Nature's youth medicines. It sold herbs exclusively. It sold Frances a special herb powder that promoted youthful regularity.

The Herb that Rejuvenated Her Digestive System. She was told to make a simple tea out of the finely cut herb known as Indian Husks. She took three cups of this tea, daily, for a week, and discovered it promoted a soothing balm-like benefit to her clogged-up digestion. She achieved a rejuvenation that promoted freedom from laxatives. She was free from the harsh carthartic slavery. Now she felt young again with Indian Husks Tea.

Benefits of Nature's Youth Medicine: This folk healer is derived from Indian psyllium, having been specially treated and washed. The resulting product is a natural hemicellulose (not a chemical methyl-cellulose) which produces a sponge-like type of active bulk which is called "activage."

No chemicals, no harsh bulk, just tiny, hungry-for-water millions of spongelike filaments actively passing through the intestinal tract and attracting to themselves the moisture and gases of the end-products of digestion.

The normally-formed waste movement is the result of this

"activage" made possible by Indian Husks, a natural herbal compound.

Helps the Dieter. Frances E. was rendered a victim of constipation because of dieting. She found that Indian Husks tea was especially beneficial because it supplied non-caloric natural bulk to fill her void caused by reduced caloric intake. She, like others on diets, are troubled with constipation because of lack of bulk through reduced food intake. But with Indian Husks, regularity is natural on any diet program. Frances E. felt and looked young again.

How Herbs May Replace Patent Medicines. In many reported situations, herbs cause a natural action on the system, replacing that of patent medicines. In the above case of Francis E., she found that her constipation was caused by the excessive use of cathartics. Whipped into action by purgatives and harsh bulk patent remedies, the intestinal tract finally fails to respond to normal stimuli. The resulting constipation is usually a combination of diarrheal movement following the laxative, followed by a period of costiveness which is only relieved by another dose of the laxative patent medicine. Herbs are unique in that they strike at the *cause* and thereby promote natural correction.

The ancients knew that herbs promote internal healing and ease the *cause* of the age-causing illness; they knew that chemical drugs relaxed the *symptoms* but did not always correct the cause. Herbs are generally non-habit forming, unlike patent medicines which often form such an addictive pattern that the body becomes enslaved to the age-causing chemicals. Herbs promote the look and feel of youth from within, while patent medicines create a false sense of security while the aging process continues. Follow the advice of the ancients—look to herbs for Nature's gift of healthy youthfulness *at any age.*

HERBAL HEALERS FOR PROLONGED YOUTH

These herbal compounds have been taken from the archives of many natural healers. A general rule of thumb is to use ¹/₂ ounce of any of these herb powders for a tea. The reported healing benefit is given first, and the reported herbal healer for prolonged youth is given afterwards:

ARTHRITIS AND RHEUMATISM. Couchgrass wood betony, prickly ash bark, sarsaparilla root, guaiacum raspings.

BACKACHE AND KIDNEY DISTRESS. Parsley, buchu, broom, wild carrot, juniper berries.

BRONCHIAL AND RESPIRATORY DISORDERS. Hyssop, comfrey root, horehound, coltsfoot leaves, liquorice juice.

COLDS AND WINTER AILMENTS. Yarrow, peppermint, elder flower, chillies.

NERVOUS AND EMOTIONAL REJUVENATION. Scullcap, mistletoe, wood betony, vervain, Peruvian bark.

BLOOD REJUVENATION. Sarsaparilla root, burdock root, sassafras bark, yellow dock root.

STOMACH AND LIVER HEALTH. Barberry bark, agrimony, centaury, meadowsweet, ginger root (crushed).

SORE THROAT AND GARGLE COMPOUND. Ragworth, red sage, chillies.

HEADACHE. Rosemary, thyme, wild thyme, wild marjoram, peppermint, lavender flowers, rose flowers, marjoram.

COUGH. Maidenhair, hart's tongue, poppy capsules, vervain, hyssop, ground ivy.

YOUTHFUL PEP TONIC. Fennel, aniseed, couchgrass, liquorice root, figs, lime flowers, hartshorn.

CHEST AND LUNGS. Marshmallow flowers, mallow flowers, coltsfoot flowers, violet flowers, mullein flowers, red poppy flowers, catsfoot flowers.

TO CLEANSE DIGESTIVE TRACT. Tansy, wormwood, wormseed (levant), chamomile.

SOOTHING YOUTH TONIC. Marshmallow flowers, mallow flowers, mullein flowers.

TO PROMOTE NORMAL BILE FLOW. Asparagus root, parsley root, celery root, fennel, butcher's broom.

TO INDUCE NATURAL PERSPIRATION. Marshmallow root,

liquorice root, orris root, ground ivy, aniseed, coltsfoot leaves, red poppy flowers, mullein.

To REJUVENATE BASIC BODY FUNCTIONS. Sassafras wood, elder flowers, red poppy flowers, borage leaves.

To PROMOTE NATURAL OXYGENATION AND EASE CONGESTION. Aniseed, fennel, caraway, coriander.

A YOUTHFUL APPETITE. Holy thistle, germander, centaury, buckbean.

SPASM CONTROL. Yarrow herb, orange flowers, valerian root.

THROAT DISORDERS. Goodsefoot, rupturewort.

DIGESTIVE-CONSTIPATION DISTRESS. Wormwood, wood betony, bugle, mountain mint, water germander, hyssop, ground ivy, yarrow, marjoram, periwinkle, rosemary, sanicle, sage, thyme, wild thyme, vervain, arnica flowers, catsfoot flowers, coltsfoot flowers.

FOR MARITAL VIGOR. Kola, damiana, saw palmetto.

HEMORRHOIDS AND PILES. Pilewort, yarrow, senna pods, poplar bark, raisins.

HIVES. Stinging nettles, yarrow, golden seal, dandelion root.

SENILE NERVE DISTRESS. Lady's slipper, vervain, valerian, scullcap, saw palmetto, raspberry leaves, peruvian bark, liverwort, kola nuts, barberry bark, mistletoe.

To EASE BODY TOXICITY. Yellow dock, queens delight.

To EASE PROBLEMS OF MIDDLE AGE. Clivers, wood betony, sanicle, chamomile.

HOW REX T. EASES HIS RECURRING HEADACHES. As an accountant, Rex T. strains his eyes. His problem is complicated because he has to hunch over a desk while he prepares accounting sheets or does long columns of figures.

Rex T. has recurring headaches that border on migraine distress. He was an aspirin "slave" which masked the symptoms but did not correct the cause. When he stopped taking aspirins or patent medicines, he was punished with a pound-

pound-pounding in his head that made him feel like exploding. His work suffered. So did his head!

A herbal pharmacy client helps him. When he complained to a client, a herbal pharmacy, he was told to make the following:

All-Natural Herb Tonic for Headache Relief

Mix 1 ounce of golden seal, 1 ounce of dandelion root and 1/2 ounce of mandrake. Steep. Drink one-half cup a half hour before each of the three daily meals.

Has Partial Relief. Rex T. enjoyed partial relief because he still took aspirins. When he discontinued his aspirins, he found that the All-Natural Herb Tonic for Headache Relief gave him merciful freedom from headaches—without drugs! Now he could work with zest. He was fortunate that his herbal pharmacy client helped him find freedom from headaches through Nature.

HERBS: NATURE'S OWN "MEDICINE" CHEST. In these natural healing grasses, we find drugless medicines, created by Nature, offered to give you the youthful health you deserve. The ancients were well aware of the youth restoration power of herbs and benefited by enjoying prolonged youthful health in an era when chemicals were unknown. Drugs and chemicals, when abused, create a corrosive aging in the system that leads to loss of youth. Herbs, on the other hand, have natural healing properties that promote youthful healing from *within* through their action upon the vital body processes. The secret of herbal healing is that it causes the body's own systems to rejuvenate and thereby offer good health at any age. Nature offers you a garden of herbs. Take them and enjoy youth!

SUMMARY:

1. Herb potions are prime sources of ingredients that promote a natural youthful feeling.

2. Establish regularity, as did Frances E., with a natural "laxative" that takes moments to prepare. Completely drugless.

3. Check the list of herbal healers and select those healing grasses for your own use as simple brews.

4. Relieve headaches and enjoy "young thoughts" and "youthful mental energy" through an All-Natural Herb Tonic. It reportedly gave Rex T. renewed mental power.

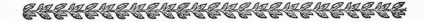

Chapter 16

Legendary Aphrodisiacs

for Those Over 40

THE legendary lovers of romantic history were sexually vigorous at "advanced" ages because they reportedly knew the secrets of blending together different all-natural potions that were said to stimulate and rejuvenate the love instinct. Many of the reputed lovers *par excellence* were well over 40 and even in their 50's and 60's, but they surpassed youngsters with their romantic powers because they used Nature to provoke the internal fountains of lovemaking splendor. They travelled the world over, searched among forgotten scrolls and parchments, talked to legendary lovers and learned the secrets of perpetual lovemaking at any age. Nearly all had found that Nature's live food juices, together with special herbs and spices, could produce a feeling of youthful vigor that helped promote the look-feel-action of youth, itself! They relied upon these potions because they were effective. They called them "aphrodisiacs" with a

175

burst of enthusiasm over the powers they bestowed. In these "aphrodisiacs" or love potions, Nature gave them the look-feel-action of youth and thereby gave them life, love, and happiness. What more could they seek?

THREE LEGENDARY HERBAL-SPICE APHRODISIACS

According to the ancients (and moderns, too), herbs and spices, when properly blended with special live food juices, have the ability to promote a feeling of rejuvenation that is equal to that of an aphrodisiac. The romantic men and women of the past long ago learned there were three special types of herbal-spice aphrodisiacs. These same spices are available, today, at most herbal pharmacies. They include:

1. *Love Spices.* These are derived from the bark, root, fruit or berry of perennial plants. Examples include cinnamon from the bark, ginger from the root, nutmeg from the fruit, and pepper from the berry.

2. *Happy Herbs.* These are the leaves of annual and perennial low-growing shrubs. Examples include basil, marjoram, tarragon, thyme, rosemary, dill weed, and chervil.

3. *Romantic Aromatic Seeds.* These are the seeds of graceful, lacy annual plants. Examples include anise, caraway, coriander, and fennel.

By using either single or combinations of these love spices, happy herbs and romantic aromatic seeds, the legendary lovers would concoct aphrodisiacs that would promote youthful well-being at any advanced age. Today, many are looking to these all-natural sources to help revive and re-stimulate the physio-reflex powers of the hormonal system so that they can enjoy life and love—to a ripe "old" age that is filled with youth.

DON JUAN'S SPECIAL LOVE POTION. The legendary Don Juan was actually a 14th century aristocratic libertine of Seville, Spain. His amorous exploits were based upon real life in which he was able to rival youngsters with his ability to charm one maiden after another, even until he was well up in his 60's and 70's. According to historians, Don Juan had a special love potion that he would prepare and drink about one hour before each seduction. Here is *Don Juan's Special Love Potion:*

> 1 cup fresh tomato juice
> 1/4 teaspoon basil leaves, crushed

Be sure to crush the basil leaves before adding to the tomato juice. Mix vigorously until the fragrance is assimilated into the tomato juice. Then sip slowly. The taste is somewhat reminiscent of licorice having a lemony, anise-like quality. Legend has it that ingredients in this special Love Potion exert a hormonal rejuvenation that promotes a feeling of romantic inclination. Don Juan may well have earned his reputation as a lover by using this all-natural aphrodisiac.

THE CASANOVA COCKTAIL. The famed lover of history, Casanova, lived from 1725–1798, and reportedly was able to provide romantic enjoyment for his female conquests even when he was over 70 years old. History says that when the end came, it was in the company of several royal ladies. At his bedside was a special aphrodisiac which he was said to take, thrice daily, for most of his life.

Here is the famed *Casanova Cocktail:*

> 1/2 teaspoon cinnamon powder
> 1/2 cup slightly steamed apple juice
> 1/2 cup grapefruit juice

Mix all ingredients vigorously and drink slowly. The legendary power of cinnamon may well be in the deep-burrowing roots of the plant. It grows to about eight feet in height before it is harvested. It often has a warm, bittersweet, and aromatic taste. In combination with the pectin power of the apple and grapefruit juices, as well as the bioflavonoid content, the reaction is like that of an aphrodisiac to the hormonal system. Casanova reportedly had this special Casanova Cocktail almost daily and would rather go without food than be without this legendary aphrodisiac. It's all-natural and this may be the secret of its unusual ability to create the look-feel-action of loving youth.

CLEOPATRA ELIXIR. The beautiful Cleopatra, as reigning Queen of Egypt, was able to use her seductive wiles upon Mark Antony and other leaders, because she would feed them a special elixir that would promote their vigor and then she would take it, herself, to be able to respond with youthful ardor. Historians say that Cleopatra was well into her 40's, yet could function with the vigor of an adolescent, because of this mystical, legendary herbal brew. She had servants prepare the Cleopatra Elixir that would be given to amorous conquests, and herself, and was thus able to gain worldwide power and renown.

Here is the legendary *Cleopatra Elixir:*

> $1/2$ teaspoon ground cloves
> $1/2$ cup papaya juice
> $1/4$ cup watermelon juice
> $1/4$ cup banana puree

If a blender is available, mix thoroughly as for a beverage. If no blender or extractor is available, then mix thoroughly with a spoon. Try to blend all ingredients. Sip slowly. Legend tells us that Cleopatra would often go on a special "fast" and subsist exclusively upon large amounts of this special Cleopatra Elixir. It reportedly gave her vigor and also promoted vigor in her partners, and she could out-rival youngsters with her ability to give and receive youthful love. The combination of cloves with the minerals and protein in the fruits works to exert a hormone-glandular revitalization that exerts a look-feel-act young ability. Cleopatra has gone down in history as an ageless lover. Today, this Cleopatra Elixir may be made in your home. Perhaps it can help you become an ageless lover in your home! Nature offers her helping hand through the Cleopatra Elixir.

THE QUEEN OF SHEBA MINT BREW. The ruler of the ancient land of Sheba, this extraordinary beauty was able to charm the wise King Solomon as well as other important men, because she had the love-making ability of a goddess. Indeed, many of her conquests expressed amazement at her stamina. They had never met her equal. With such powers, the beautiful Queen of Sheba was able to create a mighty nation that was wealthy and all-powerful. She knew there were mystical, legendary, and provocative powers in natural spices and herbs, as well as fruit and vegetable juices, and she favored these above all else. Her servants were entrusted with the secret of a special brew that she took thrice daily. It was only after one servant escaped her rule that the secret was revealed and then shared by many others who enjoyed a feeling of "perpetual" youth with this romantic brew.

Here is the legendary *Queen Of Sheba Mint Brew:*

> $1/2$ teaspoon crushed peppermint or spearmint spice
> $1/4$ cup carrot juice
> $1/4$ cup potato juice
> $1/4$ cup cabbage juice

The juices should be freshly prepared. Mix the crushed mint in with the juices and stir vigorously. Sip slowly. About one cup, taken three times daily, reportedly provided this legendary beauty of Sheba with the power to win over the affection of a retinue of influential men. Today, these all-natural juices may be enjoyed by everyone. The "magic" power may well be in the mint which is a hardy perennial plant; its essential oil has been known to produce a hormone-like effect that whips up the glandular network and promotes a revival power that promotes a love of life and a life of love. The Queen of Sheba guarded this Mint Brew formula with secrecy. Happily, it is available today.

PARSLEY: THE HERB OF YOUNG LOVERS AT ALL AGES

Parsley is a low-growing biennial plant belonging to the celery family. The nativity of this popular "love-creating" herb dates back to the third century, B.C. During the times when Greece and Rome flourished, many tired soldiers, businessmen, and weary wives, would visit the local herbalist and obtain parsley for use in soups, broths and stews. They extolled the love-making virtues of this particular herb.

Europeans Feared Its Aphrodisiac Powers. The legendary love-producing powers of parsley spread throughout Europe and so alarmed many of the people that it was not accepted there until the thirteenth century. It is said that in 1548, a shepherd secretly brought in the first plants to be cultivated on his little farm in Sardinia, a small island in the Mediterranean, west of Italy. Here, parsley plants flourished and were sold in secret to a select few who reportedly derived such aphrodisiac powers that they had to resist taking this herb. Gradually, the cultivation was increased and it was soon flourishing throughout Europe.

Vigor Power in Leaves. The vigor-producing power of this legendary herb may well be in its leaves. These are rich in Vitamins A and C and also iron, iodine, manganese, and copper. But more important, when parsley leaves are crushed, a unique oil is released that helps create a rejuvenation power to the glandular-hormonal network. Since lovemaking vigor is often related to hormone health, the parsley "oil" may well be the legendary secret of its ability to create the look-feel-action of youth at all ages.

How to Use Parsley: Mix 1/2 teaspoon in soups such as minestrone, vegetable, beef, or chicken broth. The heat of the soup helps release many of the pungent powers in the dried leaves of the parsley herb, thereby enabling them to enter into the metabolism and life processes of the digestive system. The "oil" as well as the nutrients then work to promote a feeling of rejuvenation and well-being that leads to a feeling of romantic youth.

Parsley Potent Potion: Legend tells us that the Sardinian shepherd was well up in his 60's when he began planting parsley in his own garden. He was worried about losing his lovemaking powers, especially since he had wed a girl in her very early 20's. (Her father owned a large adjoining farm and it was hoped that the aging shepherd would be able to acquire it because of his marriage. He wanted to enjoy his remaining years in comfortable luxury which would be possible with this rich soil farm.) But the Sardinian shepherd feared that if he could not act young with his young wife, he would lose her as well as the chance of obtaining her father's farm. So he prepared this special *Parsley Potent Potion:*

 $^1/_2$ teaspoon crushed parsley
 $^1/_2$ cup freshly squeezed lettuce juice
 $^1/_2$ cup tomato juice
 1 tablespoon beet juice
 2 tablespoons radish juice

Mix all ingredients thoroughly together. Drink one glass before breakfast, a second glass before lunch, a third glass before dinner.

The unique benefit of this special Parsley Potent Potion is in the amino acid content of the beets and radishes and the minerals in the lettuce and tomato. Together with the "oil" and released vitamins of the parsley, there is a special enzymatic action that reportedly whips up the hormonal structure and promotes glandular function. The benefit here is in the feeling of supercharged vigor that enables one to enjoy the reported aphrodisiac powers of this special Parsley Potent Potion.

History tells us that the Sardinian shepherd used this secret potion and was able to become the father of children, even when he was well beyond the age of 60. He eventually acquired the adjoining farm, became prosperous and lived to a ripe "young" age that neared the century mark. The legend is that when his demise came, he was about to become a father as he neared the eleventh decade of his life. He had a glass of Parsley Potent Potion beside him at the end. Someone secreted it away, tasted it, and was able to prepare the formula with the help of local alchemists. It had served well as an all-natural aphrodisiac!

THE EXECUTIVE FEELS LIKE A
BRIDEGROOM AGAIN

Ralph T., an over-40 executive, found that while his business was prospering, his romantic life was showing a downward descent. Undoubtedly, the nervous pressure and tension of business did drain out his energy and siphon off his romantic abilities. But even during a vacation, away from office responsibilities, Ralph T. found himself embarrassed by marital weakness. His wife felt rightfully nervous and upset. Both disliked the use of chemical drugs that were said to promote a feeling of well-being. It was his wife who took the problem to a local herbal pharmacist who suggested the use of a legendary herb known as the damiana plant. (The pharmaceutical or Latin name is *Turnera diffusa*.)

This particular herb is reported to have aphrodisiac powers. It is said to have a general and beneficial action on the body's organs while serving as a stimulant to the nervous system. Because it is all-natural, it may be used for helping to revive the dormant powers bestowed by Nature. Its leaves are used to create extract of damian. Several drops, mixed with a glass of fresh fruit juice, help stimulate and renourish the lovemaking glandular system.

Ralph T. took this special legendary elixir for several days. He found that he felt such a resurgence of vigor, it was like being on a second honeymoon. Small wonder he called it a special Bridegroom Love Elixir. It gave Ralph T. the vigor of a bridegroom and now, even with increased business worries, he could act like a bridegroom on a honeymoon. Nature gave second youth to this 40-plus man.

Most herbal pharmacies have extract of damian. Mix several drops in a glass of fresh fruit juice, drink thrice daily, and give Nature a chance to give you the second best 40 years of your life!

HELP YOURSELF TO LEGENDARY LOVEMAKING POWER WITH NATURE'S HERBS. By using the wide variety of natural herbs and spices, in combination with fresh live juices, you help feed your glandular-hormonal system the supercharged vitamins, minerals, amino acids, and enzymes that work in harmony to create a look-feel-act young again power. Nature meant for man and woman to enjoy love to a ripe "young" age. Nature provided the working materials for stimulating the love processes with her garden of herbs, spices, and plants. Use them and reap the harvest of legendary lovemaking power—at any age. When you love others and are loved by others, you then enjoy a youthful happiness that is brimming with health and beauty. Through Nature's potions, you are given this reward—you are able to give love and be loved in return. That, if anything, is the secret of the look and feel of youth.

IN SUMMARY:

1. Aphrodisiacs are legendary love potions that promote the feeling of romance in men and women at all ages.
2. Three legendary herbal-spice aphrodisiacs are available today at herb pharmacies.
3. Don Juan's Special Love Potion earned him his scandalous reputation.
4. The Casanova Cocktail made him an international lover.
5. The Cleopatra Elixir was a powerhouse of aphrodisiacs.
6. The all-natural Queen of Sheba Mint Brew made her an ageless lover.
7. The Parsley Potent Potion is a miracle of lovemaking power.
8. Enjoy a second honeymoon at any age with the all-natural Bridegroom Love Elixir.

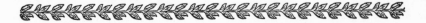

Chapter 17

How to Drink Your Way to a

Youthful Slim-Trim Waistline

GERALDINE fought the battle of the bulge with special diet programs, group therapy weight reducing clubs, expensive slenderizing salons, monotonous exercises, and just about everything else that came along. Her latest hope for achieving a youthful figure was to join a jogging group. This so exhausted Geraldine F. that she developed leg cramps, chronic fatigue, and a feeling of vertigo. She was still "unpleasingly plump" and had to keep changing her wardrobe to obtain larger sizes every few months. Geraldine F. liked to eat food and was unable to find satisfaction with any special reducing programs. She still had a craving for satisfying her runaway appetite. She sighed, resigned to her big bulges and ever-increasing girth. At age 44, she soon looked like 66. She felt much older than that. All because of her increasing waistline and uncontrollable appetite.

HOW A FRESH FRUIT DRINK HELPED TAME A "WILD

APPETITE." It was her plump teen-age daughter who showed Geraldine F. the way to use an all-natural beverage with one inexpensive fruit and help tame her "wild appetite." When Geraldine F. overheard her plump daughter talking on the telephone, lamenting that she did not want to be a "fat slob" like her mother and would try this special drink, the mother experienced an emotional shock. Geraldine F. never thought her daughter regarded her a "fat slob" but realized perhaps it was true. She certainly did make a poor image in her unsightly bulging clothes. She then listened and heard that her daughter had been given a special tasty drink that was all-natural and helped put the brakes on a runaway appetite.

Geraldine's daughter had been given this simple recipe by a dietician in school. It consisted of just two ingredients. Combined together with a blender, or by using a wire whisk to mix together, it acted as a stop gap to the bottomless appetite of compulsive eaters such as Geraldine and even her young daughter.

How TO MAKE A SLIM-YOUNG BEVERAGE. In a tall glass, mash two bananas with skimmed milk. Blend together thoroughly. Drink this *before* you partake of any meal. If possible, drink *two* glasses of this Slim-Young Beverage in place of a meal. The combination of nutrients in the Slim-Young Beverage helps promote a feeling of satisfaction that takes the edge off the appetite and helps control an eating urge.

How the Slim-Young Beverage Made Geraldine Look Young Again. Geraldine F. would drink one glass of the Slim-Young Beverage before each of her meals. She would also drink a glass whenever she felt the urge to eat something. The benefit in controlling the appetite is that in the raw banana, there are "full," rather than "empty" calories that help ease the urge to eat. The banana contains beneficial Vitamins A, B-complex, niacin and many essential minerals.

Helps Fill Up without Filling Out. The skimmed milk has vitamins and minerals that act as *jet-stream activators* upon the banana to help provide pectin and delicate fiber network to add to gastro-intestinal bulk. This promotes easy digestion. This unique action helps you fill up on "low calories" without filling out! The distinctive mellow flavor of the Slim-Young Beverage provides a comfortable feeling and helps promote cheerfulness, even on a low-fat diet. The action of the carbohydrate in the banana as a protein-sparer is helpful in maintaining the nutritional status while enabling the person to slim down.

Promotes Youthful Slenderness without Drugs. Geraldine F. found that by controlling her appetite with the Slim-Young Beverage, she could give up her appetite depressing drugs (they often made her dizzy), and look to Nature for slimming down. This beverage, with the banana, offered highly digestible and absorbable carbohydrates, essential vitamins, minerals, and enzymes, and had a high satiety value, with a "staying" power equalled by few other foods, except those containing considerable amounts of fat. Where drugs had to be used to control the urge to eat fat foods, now this all-natural beverage could be used to help promote youthful slenderness.

Looks Younger than Her Daughter. It took several months of appetite-control and the Slim-Young Beverage to help trim off unsightly age-causing bulges and put back a youthful shape and firm figure. Soon, Geraldine F. looked younger than her daughter who could not resist constant snacks and remained unpleasingly plump. Geraldine F. solved her overweight problem with the Slim-Young Beverage that controlled the wild appetite and made her look and feel young. When a new neighbor thought that Geraldine F. was the younger sister of the plump daughter, the mother knew Nature had, indeed, made her young again. If only her daughter would cooperate with Nature!

HOW LIVE FOOD JUICES HELP PROMOTE A YOUTHFUL FIGURE

Live raw juices often promote a happy feeling of satisfaction and comfortable "fullness" that eases the urge to eat to excess. Many live food juices are prime sources of vitamins, minerals, enzymes, and amino acids, and can be used to promote nutritional satisfaction while on a low-calorie food program.

Heated Liquids Promote Feeling of Stomach Fullness. Heated liquids create a feeling of tissue expansiveness that gives the satisfaction of stomach fullness. Many have found that by heating raw juices to the simmering level, and sipping slowly, the benefit is an appetite-controlled "stomach fullness" that eases the compulsion to eat to excess.

Protein-Rich Vegetable Juices to Replace Fat-Rich Foods. Benjamin U. was overweight at the age of 46. His heavy stomach bulge rivalled that of his wrinkled chin bulge. He had "triple chins" that sagged and gave him the look and feel of someone much older.

Benjamin's problem was that he needed a lot of protein to feed his skin tissues and cells; on a low-fat and low-protein reducing program, his chin became flabby and his stomach started to sag. At a local gym, someone said he had "accordian-like" skin. He could not reduce without developing the unsightly skin sag that made him look and feel much older. A nutritionist prepared this following chart which shows how protein-rich vegetable juices are able to replace fat-rich animal-protein foods.

Note that many of the vegetable juices have a greater percentage of protein than the listed animal foods. These are based on equal-calorie portions:

LOW PROTEIN PERCENTAGE IN MEATS	HIGH PROTEIN PERCENTAGE IN VEGETABLE JUICES
19%—Choice club steak	Spinach—33%
19%—Porterhouse Steak	Asparagus—30%
18%—Prime T-Bone Steak	Broccoli—30%
25%—Corned Beef (medium fat)	Brussels Sprouts—29%
20%—Lamb Loin (broiled)	Kale—29%
17%—Rib Lamb Chop	Lentils—29%
18%—Spare Ribs (braised)	Collard Greens—27%
7%—Pork-Fat, raw, edible	Cauliflower—26%
16%—Cured Pork (country style)	Cabbage (Savoy)—25%
19%—Sausage (country style)	Swiss Chard—25%
17%—Deviled Ham	Green Peas—24%
18%—Frankfurter (all meat)	Lettuce—18%
20%—Bacon (well-fried & drained)	Radish—17%
18%—Prime Rib Roast	Celery—16%

How 14 PROTEIN-RICH JUICES HELPED PROMOTE YOUTH-
FUL SLENDERNESS. From the above list of 14 high-protein and
low-calorie vegetables, a variety of fresh juices could be
prepared that would help promote tissue tonus and firm
skin-texture on a low-fat but high-protein program.

Many of the preceding 14 vegetables may be prepared as
raw juices. Many others may be prepared in the form of a
heated broth or a thick "stew" that helps promote a feeling of
satiety and enables the overweight person to feel comfortably
fed on a low-calorie but high-protein meatless fare.

Benjamin U.'s Program:

1. *Young Again Breakfast Tonic.* He would prepare a fresh
raw juice made of lettuce, radishes and celery. This helped
give him a supercharging of amino acids that controlled his
appetite until noon.

2. *Appetite-Control Protein Punch.* At lunchtime, Benjamin
U. was tempted with so many high-calorie dishes. To help
control his craving and to help him feel satisfied with lesser
portions, he prepared a special Appetite-Control Protein
Punch made of spinach, cabbage, and cauliflower. These three
raw vegetable juices were prime sources of amino acids that
joined with minerals to maintain a unique "water balance" in
the glandular system to ease the urge to eat, and to help give
Benjamin U. a comfortable feeling of satisfaction.

3. *Slender Juice.* At dinnertime, faced with the traditional
and often habitual heavy meal, Benjamin U. was able to say
"no" to extra-fat meals because he prepared a warm broth
made of lentils, asparagus, and green peas. These three
vegetables provided him with valuable amino acids that
entered into the bloodstream, created a "stopgap" action
through hormonal influence on the various glands, and helped
ease the compulsion to eat. True, he did eat his dinner, but in
smaller portions. The warm Slender Juice helped curb the
appetite and bring down his waistline.

Five Months to Make Him Grow Younger. It took only five
months of the three-step program before Benjamin U. looked
and felt younger. He soon passed up extra-rich foods, extra-

rich desserts and snacks, and found that by interchanging any of the 14 protein-rich juices listed above, he could enjoy a variety of taste satisfactions. He lost his paunch and chins. He still had a slight sag to his skin, but with healthful massage and exercise, he hoped to "melt" this condition too. Soon, Benjamin U. looked youthfully slender. No longer was he the spectacle of derision by so-called friends and onlookers. Live raw juices had helped him grow younger.

How a "Nature-Sweet Raw Juice" Helped Tame a Compulsive Appetite. Adele R. was a statistical typist at a large company. She sat most of the time and this lack of exercise meant that excess calories became stored as fat. She looked much older because of her heavy girth, not to mention the unsightly bulges that could not be disguised with the latest of fashions. She could not control her compulsive appetite and she realized she was passed up for parties and social functions because she looked much older with her heavy weight. Still, her problem was more than just lack of activity. It was her compulsive appetite. She had to eat and eat and eat and snack and snack and snack. This added unsightly age-causing pounds.

Nature-Sweet Raw Juice Soothes Eating-Urge. An examination showed that Adele R. had a mild condition of hypoglycemia or low blood sugar. Her metabolism was such that it craved sugar and this hormonal "tug of war" gave her a glandular urge to continue eating. The key to appetite-control was in stabilizing her blood sugar and thereby controlling the urge to eat. She was told to prepare:

Nature-Sweet Raw Juice. Mix one-half cup of grape juice, one-half cup of apple juice, and two mashed bananas. Blend together. Drink one Nature-Sweet Raw Juice *before* each meal. If necessary, drink one Nature-Sweet Raw Juice whenever the eating urge strikes.

Benefits: The natural sugars in grapes and apples combine with the fruit sugar of the bananas. When absorbed into the system, the blood sugar concentration is gradually maintained in the bloodstream to create a slowly-released carbohydrate action to control a compulsive appetite.

RAW JUICE TAMES APPETITE AND TAMES FIGURE. This special Nature-Sweet Raw Juice worked to help tame Adele's appetite and, in turn, rewarded her with a slimmer figure. Soon, she could wear smaller sized clothes, looked refreshingly young and was much sought after for dates. Even though she still has little exercise, she is able to maintain a slimmer figure because she controls her appetite through satisfied blood sugar levels. She drinks the Nature-Sweet Raw Juice regularly and looks-feels-acts younger than ever before!

HOW TO ENJOY TASTY FOODS AND LIQUIDS WHILE SLIMMING DOWN

To look and feel young, it is essential to have a youthfully slim figure or physique. Here are several suggestions on how to enjoy tasty foods and liquids in a corrective food program that will help give you the slim look and feel of youth:

1. Dairy beverages should be fat-free. Select skimmed milk in place of whole milk.

2. To promote a feeling of satiety, use *hot* liquids that create an expansive satisfaction in the digestive system. Use beef or chicken broths *after* the fat has been skimmed off. Use bouillon cubes for clear soup.

3. Replace weight-causing salad dressings with lemon juice, tomato juice with a sprinkle of apple cider vinegar.

4. Vegetable juices are especially beneficial since they give a "fill-up" feeling that does not require the use of calorie-high salad oil dressings.

5. Fruit juices should be freshly prepared at home if possible, or all-natural, *without* the addition of any sugars.

6. Alcoholic beverages are high in calories and add age-causing pounds. Try this Natural Non-Alcoholic Cocktail: Mix 1/4 cup orange juice, 4 tablespoons apple cider vinegar, 1 tablespoon lemon juice, 1/2 cup seasonal berry juice, and 1/4 cup papaya juice. Use a cinnamon stick for a swizzle. Stir vigorously. Ice cubes may be used to complete the effect. The blending of tart-piquant flavors of this Natural Non-Alcoholic

Cocktail, together with the sweet, helps satisfy the taste buds and give the feeling of a tavern brew.

7. Begin each meal with a fresh vegetable juice. This helps "fill up" to help control the urge to eat voluminously. For compulsive eaters, beverages offer a helpful means of controlling the urge and giving a stomach-satisfying feeling of fullness.

ENJOY EXTENDED YOUTH WITH A HEALTHFULLY SLIM BODY. Science tells us that youthfulness can be extended with a healthfully youthful body that is slim and trim. By low-calorie eating and the nutritious benefits of live food juices, you can help yourself to youth with a slim-trim waistline. A "young weight" helps you look and feel young!

IN REVIEW:

1. A Slim-Young Beverage helped Geraldine tame her appetite.
2. Special protein-rich vegetable juices ease the requirement for protein-fat-rich meats.
3. Benjamin U. slimmed down by following a 3-step program that gave him vegetable protein without excess fat.
4. Select any of the listed 14 vegetables to obtain liquid protein.
5. A Nature-Sweet Raw Juice tamed Adele's compulsive appetite.
6. Just seven steps help you enjoy foods and liquids while slimming down.
7. Ease up on fattening alcoholic beverages with the special Natural Non-Alcoholic Cocktail.

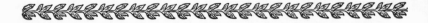

Chapter 18

How to Help Recharge Your Arteries

and Veins for Youthful Energy

Y OU look and feel as young as your arteries! If you can keep your arterial-venous network in a smooth and elastic condition, you have hopes for a long and healthy lifespan that radiates the joy of youthfulness at all ages. One way to help boost the smooth resiliency of the system of arteries and veins is to help control problems of cholesterol which lead to arteriosclerosis or aging of the arteries and body. Many people have reported that by following special liquid eating guides, they have successfully recharged their arterial-venous networks and enjoyed youthful energy.

Accumulated Fats Predispose to Hardening of the Arteries. This is not a heart condition, in the strict sense of the word, but a disorder of the arteries. It is caused by fatty deposits containing cholesterol which thicken the artery walls, thus choking off space in the arteries needed by the blood for youthful circulation. If this happens in the big arteries that feed blood to the heart, it creates an impediment to blood flow. If it occurs during severe activity, when the blood requirement increases, it will bring about heart distress signals such as chest pressure pains and angina. This problem is said to occur in 3 out of every 10 persons between the ages of 40 and 50; 5 out of every 10 persons between 50 and 60; 8 out of 10 between 60 and 70, and 9 out of 10 of all those over 70. The problem here is that this so-called "aging illness" is increasing among the 40-year olds and is being seen in increasing amounts among those under the age of 40. This calls for attention to help prevent the onset of premature aging caused by accumulated fats that cling to the arterial-venous network of the body.

HOW A NATURAL JUICE RECHARGES THE ARTERIES WITH YOUTH

Harold O. developed severe angina pains as well as such stiffening of the limbs that he was unable to work as a check out clerk at the large supermarket. His fingers trembled, were stiff and unmanageable. He could hardly make up packages. He developed such nervous tremors that he dropped packages and broke many of the products that required handling in the supermarket. At age 50, he thought he was finished because a company doctor said he had cholesterol problems and a mild form of arteriosclerosis. He was fortunate in having a doctor who believed in natural methods of internal cleansing. The doctor prepared this special three-ingredient natural juice:

The "Young Vigor" Tonic. Mix one tablespoon lecithin powder into one glass of tomato juice. Add one tablespoon brewer's yeast. Stir vigorously. Drink one glass before each of the three daily meals. A fourth glass, about an hour before bedtime, is beneficial.

The Artery-Washing Power of the "Young Vigor" Tonic. The "magic" power here may well be in the three ingredients that work harmoniously within the system. Here is what they do within the body:

1. *Lecithin.* This is a bland, water-soluble, grandular powder made from de-fatted soya beans. It is a phosphatide which means that it is a youth-promoting constitutent of all living cells. Physicians have found that lecithin is able to remove the cholesterol "plaques" that are deposited on artery walls. This all-natural ingredient helps dissolve and remove the atherosclerotic plaques from the artery walls. Another power-house of energy lies in lecithin's ability to increase the gamma globulin content of the blood proteins. These gamma globulins are known to be associated with Nature's protective force against the attacks of various body infections. It is this youthful energizing power of lecithin that has made it so essential for helping to wash the arterial-venous network.

2. *Tomato juice.* Here is a vegetable that is a prime source of the B-complex and C vitamins which work to energize the lecithin power. An alkaline vegetable because of its high mineral content, it helps neutralize excessively acid stomach distress and promotes assimilation of essential artery-washing nutrients. It has a magnetic action upon the lecithin and propels it throughout the bloodstream to perform its youthful recharging power.

3. *Brewer's yeast.* This is the tiny cell from the yeast plant. This nutritional powerhouse consists of vitamins, minerals, and amino acids. It is regarded a veritable treasure of youth-promoting nutrients. It works with lecithin and promotes the ability to manufacture the esterases enzymes or activators that aid in the metabolizing of fats. Brewer's yeast with lecithin and tomato juice, in this "Young Vigor" Tonic help create a self-cleansing action that promotes an arterial recharging and rejuvenation feeling for extended health.

How Harold O. Enjoys New Lease on Life with "Young Vigor" Tonic. The supermarket worker followed the program for look-feel-act young; he eliminated artificial "fluff" foods, synthetic foods, and emphasized natural foods. He took this "Young Vigor" Tonic four times daily. It took several months before he experienced a renewed flexibility of his joints and could return to work with supple and youthful fingers and joints. He was given a new lease on life through natural liquids.

HOW SEED OILS PROMOTE A CHOLESTEROL-WASHING BENEFIT

Doctors report that seed oils are able to help wash off the cholesterol deposits that lead to a condition of clogged arteries and veins. The secret ingredient in seed oils is that of Vitamin E which doctors report as being most beneficial in helping to prevent, correct and relieve the problem of atherosclerotic plaques upon the arterial-venous network of the body.

Seed Oils Work While You Sleep. Doctors report that seed oils, with their Vitamin A as well as Vitamin E content, create a self-washing benefit while you sleep! Both of these nutrients are fat-soluble. When carried in solution in cholesterol, they bring about changes in that fat. Both work to prevent the rancidity and the production of hydrogen peroxide. In turn, this benefit helps prevent and relieve age-causing atherosclerotic plaques, while you sleep!

Natural Sources Of Seed Oils. Good natural sources include wheat germ oil, cottonseed oil, soya oil, safflower seed oil, corn oil, peanut oil, and olive oil.

YOUTH-BUILDING NIGHTCAP. One good way to get Vitamin E is in the form of this special and tasty Youth-Building Nightcap. Add two tablespoons of wheat germ flakes to one cup of soya milk (which is a prime source of lecithin), and add one tablespoon of mineral-rich honey for blood rejuvenation. Drink about one hour before retiring. When the body is at rest in sleep, the ingredients of this Youth-Building Nightcap go to work to help energize the arterial-venous network so that you should awaken with a feeling of abundant youth and flexibility.

HOW PLANT JUICE PROMOTES "YOUNG AGAIN" ARTERIES. Good plant juice sources of Vitamin E include dandelion leaves, kale, green leafy tops of leeks, mustard leaves, nasturtium leaves, nettle leaves, parsley leaves, soybeans, spinach, sweet potato, and turnip leaves. If you can run these plants through a juicer and drink the liquid foods, you will be giving your arteries a powerful "young again" supply of Vitamin E.

Special Health Tip: Vitamin E is more concentrated in the leaves of plants than in the roots or stems. It is more potent in green leaves than in pale leaves; it is more concentrated in large or mature leaves than in small or immature leaves.

THE LIQUID FOOD THAT EXTENDED YOUTHFUL LIFE

A medical journal tells of three physicians who treated 28 prematurely aging patients who were victims of myocardial infarction or heart trouble; they also had high blood cholesterol levels. The patients were divided into controlled groups. Put on a special low animal fat diet, their blood cholesterol decreased. But a more remarkable arterial-venous energizing and youthfication was noted when the doctors prepared this special elixir:

Nu-Youth Liquid Food. Combine safflower oil, plus pyridoxine (one of the B-complex vitamins) and sterols (plant juice from the above list). Mix in a fresh vegetable juice. Combine with 20 milligrams of Vitamin E. Drink one cup of this Nu-Youth Liquid Food daily, with each meal, and one more at bedtime.

Rewards In Extended Life. The doctors reported that this special Nu-Youth Liquid Food, in combination with low animal fat intake, successfully lowered the blood cholesterol of the patients who were rewarded with an extended life, without arteriosclerosis.

Benefits: Both Vitamins B-complex and E, together with the unsaturated fatty acids in the plant juice, worked to act as an anti-oxidant, to spare body requirement of oxygen, and promote a lowering of cholesterol content in the blood. The doctors reported that the arteries and veins could be recharged with youthful energy through the proper use of liquid foods and the prescribed all-natural Nu-Youth Liquid Food.

Other Factors that Influence Arterial Youth. Emotional stress, evidenced in situations when pressure is high at work, or family difficulties become irritating, can also cause a rise in the level of blood cholesterol. Excess calories from either fats or carbohydrates and insufficient physical activity will lead to a weight gain and unhealthy rise in blood cholesterol that threatens the youth of the arteries. A program for melting of cholesterol should include natural liquid foods, tranquility, moderate prescribed exercises, and corrective solid foods with decreasing amounts of high-fat foods. Many physicians in supervised medical programs have been able to restore youth to the arterial-venous networks of patients with an all-around alliance with Nature.

WHY HEALTHY ARTERIES ARE THE PIPELINES OF YOUTH

The arteries are specially constructed elastic pipelines of youth. They are made of *three* layers:

1. The outer protective coat carries the nerves and blood vessels supplying the artery itself.

2. The middle layer is the thickest and is composed of elastic and muscular fibers.

3. The inner coat is a thin, smooth lining.

As these arteries branch throughout the body, they become smaller and thinner so that the finest ones are thread-like, with very delicate walls that permit body solutions to pass in and out. The youthful processes of the body depend upon healthy arteries that permit functioning of a healthy and youthful bloodstream.

How Oils Help Ease the Aging Threat of Arteriosclerosis. Unsaturated oils are reported as having the power to act as "blocking agents" to keep harmful fats out of the blood. The term *unsaturated* is used by doctors to mean that the fat molecule still has room to add additional molecules onto its structure. Therefore, it is lighter in weight and more easily handled by the blood, reducing the age-causing threat of arteriosclerosis.

Suggested Oils: These are so-called "soft" fats—those that are liquid at room temperature. They include most vegetable oils, such as olive, cottonseed, corn, soya, peanut, etc. The one exception is coconut oil which is saturated, even though it is liquid. Other free-flowing "soft" fats include wheat germ oil, lecithin oil, rice germ oil, to name a few. These are reportedly good oils in the program to ease the age-causing threat of arteriosclerosis.

GARDEN OF YOUTH SALAD DRESSING. Miriam J., a young-looking clothes designer, found new flexibility in her limbs when she prepared a special salad dressing. She would mix four tablespoons of wheat germ oil, four tablespoons of soya oil together with one heaping tablespoon of lecithin. She would use this Garden of Youth Salad Dressing on a bowl of fresh raw vegetables. This introduced a powerhouse of Vitamin E to her system. When she followed a special low animal fat program, she was able to control her cholesterol level, and enjoy a youthful flexibility of her limbs that increased her work output and general outlook on life. She felt young again with her daily Garden of Youth Salad Dressing.

HOW LECITHIN PROMOTED ARTERIAL REJUVENATION IN TWO "OVER-40" PATIENTS

A doctor who used a liquid eating guide for patients, reported that two of his patients responded with dramatic youth-restoration benefits when they used lecithin in their corrective programs. He reported these two cases:

1. Mrs. U., a 45-year old housewife, was ashamed of the flat plaques of yellowish hue that appeared on her skin caused by fatty deposits. She put lecithin into her eating program, and the doctor reports that these age-causing plaques soon disappeared. "Mrs. U. was more delighted with what she saw

happening in the mirror than with the idea that the same thing might be going on with the fatty deposits inside her arteries," says the doctor.

2. John Y., a baker in his middle 40's, suffered so acutely from angina (chest pain caused by choked off blood supply to the heart muscle) that he could not work. He also had many yellowish brown plaques under his eyes, where fatty deposits appeared. The doctor reports taking John's cholesterol level and finding it to be abnormally high. The doctor put John on a low-cholesterol, low-fat program but emphasized the use of lecithin in cocktails (fruit or vegetable juices), sprinkled over salads, or taken in soya milks. The doctor reports that within a few months, John Y. was able to return to work, free of anginal pain. His cholesterol level was admirably lowered and the fatty plaques (known as *xanthalasma*) vanished from his face.

Lecithin, a powerhouse of artery-washing ingredients, is reported as being vital for helping to recharge the arteries and veins for youthful energy.

HOW AN "ENERGY ELIXIR" PROMOTES INTERNAL REJUVENATION

Instead of the habitual "coffee break," Richard E., an office manager, uses a special Energy Elixir which he prepares in the morning, at home, in a thermos bottle. Richard E. mixed these ingredients together:

> 2 tablespoons powdered brewer's yeast
> 1/2 cup skimmed milk
> 1/2 cup soya milk
> 1 tablespoon organic honey

Richard E. has found that when he drinks one cup of this Energy Elixir, he experiences an overall rejuvenation and "tingling" of the extremities that promote a feeling of invigoration and youth.

Benefits of Energy Elixir: The powerhouse of the B-complex vitamins works with the minerals and enzymes in the milk and honey to help nourish the arterial-venous network. In particular, this Energy Elixir contains three specific B-complex vitamins—choline, inositol, and pyridoxine. These three work together to ease and control hardening of the arteries by dispersing globules of fat in much the same way as lecithin. The ingredients in the Energy Elixir break up blood fat into tiny globules which can then be easily assimilated. The cholesterol level and age-causing arteriosclerosis is thereby checked or controlled through this all-natural liquid food. Richard E. thinks, works, looks, feels, and acts young with this simple yet effective liquid food.

How a "Yeast Cocktail" Stimulates Internal Revitalization. Eloise E. is a saleswoman who has to be on her feet most of the day. She needs an alert mind as much as she does an alert body. When she found herself developing stiff fingers, painful knees, and aching joints that worsened with the change of the weather, as well as a recurring backache that gave her a stooped gait, she sought medical help. Her physician told her to correct her eating fare, to include more natural raw foods, and to cut down on animal or "hard" fats. This helped control her situation, but she still felt "sluggish inside." The health nutritionist suggested this special:

"Yeast Cocktail": Mix four tablespoons of powdered brewer's yeast in fruit juice. Season with honey to taste. Drink one glass, at least three or four times daily.

Benefits: This "Yeast Cocktail" was rich in 17 different vitamins, including the entire B-family group. It was also rich in good protein and minerals yet it had only one per cent fat. The benefit here is that this Yeast Cocktail was able to feed the nervous system, soothe the gastrointestinal system, and also help in the metabolism of starches and fats. This reduced the excess cholesterol and restored supple flexibility to Eloise's joints. She could again walk straight and could use her fingers with the agility of a young girl. This simple, yet potently youth-building "Yeast Cocktail" stimulated her sluggish internal systems and brought about needed revitalization.

How Liquid Foods Help Promote "Second-Youth Arteries." Liquid foods and raw juices are prime sources of unsaturated, non-processed and natural substances that are able to become speedily metabolized to then promote arterial cleansing. In solids, the metabolization rate is much slower and there is a release and coating of waste substances that may contribute to the formation of deposits upon the arterial and vein system. Liquid foods have another unique youth-restoration benefit. They play an important role in thyroid function by their ability to combine with freely available iodine and release it slowly. This helps promote normal cholesterol metabolism. Liquid foods thus encourage a self-cleansing autolysis action and thereby promote "second youth arteries" with resilient elasticity and function.

SUMMARY:

1. Enjoy the feeling of youth with a "washed" arterial structure.
2. Harold O. responded well to the "Young Vigor" Tonic made with three simple store-purchased ingredients.
3. Seed oils promote a cholesterol-washing benefit that works while you sleep. Enjoy a "Youth-Building Nightcap."
4. Plant juices promote "young again" arteries.
5. The Nu-Youth Liquid Food was used to extend youthful life in patients.
6. Healthy arteries are the pipelines of youthfulness.
7. Two patients reportedly enjoyed arterial rejuvenation by using lecithin, a natural food.
8. A simply prepared "Energy Elixir" helped boost vitality by helping to correct cholesterol conditions.
9. A "Yeast Cocktail" gave a woman a second chance for a "new youthfulness."

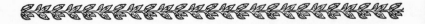

Chapter 19

Your One-Day "All Liquid"

Youth-Restoration Program

To help release your locked-in potential for the look
and feel of youth, controlled fasting is an historic, time-tested
folk healer that has been used ever since recorded history.
Controlled fasting in which you partake solely of certain
liquids, is especially beneficial since it relaxes-rests-
rejuvenates the basic sense systems of the mind and body.
Just as the body needs rest during sleep, so do the internal
organisms require a day of rest from their often over-worked
responsibilities of metabolism-assimilation-respiration. It is
through an "all liquid" day of controlled fasting that you give
your internal organisms the rest they deserve. You are then
rewarded with a healthier, refreshed internal organism that is
reflected in the look and glow of youthfulness on the outside.

REWARDS OF A SUCCESSFUL YOUTH-RESTORATION FAST.
During one day of controlled fasting on fresh raw and living
juices, the body organism enjoys reconstitution; the enervat-

ed nervous system is given a chance to rest, no longer required to strenuously participate in various processes. With such a benefit, elimination of metabolic waste substances tends to increase because of more youthful function. To the extent that enervation is corrected, elimination improved, and the secretory and assimilative capacities corrected, there are resultant benefits of fasting.

Controlled "All Liquid" Fasting Melts Away Burdensome Weight. The necessary food supply to maintain vital organic structures and the essential functions during the fast is derived from the body tissue reserves or the stored up fat deposits. Therefore, excess fat and other tissue encumbrances are used as a source of food. There is weight loss with a controlled "all liquid" fasting program. Many who are troubled by obesity would do well to look to this ancient folk healer for slimming down without pills or drugs.

Live Food Juices Help Wash Away Internal Wastes. Live food juices that are consumed during a one-day controlled fasting program, work best without interference of solids eaten at the same time. They are able to cause a self-cleansing of accumulated debris from the internal organs. This is a form of cleansing and detoxification of the sludge-covered organs so that the entire body enjoys this cleansing benefit from drinking live food juices.

HOW LIQUID FASTING REJUVENATES FIVE HEALTH SYSTEMS

To enjoy the look and feel of youth, the five valuable health systems should be in tip-top shape. Controlled liquid fasting works upon these five valuable youth-restoring systems as follows:

1. *Supercharges Metabolism with Youthful Vitality.* Live food juices help to nourish the process of metabolism. This is the system that converts food into energy. Nutrients in raw juices provide electrical energy to the metabolic system to give youthful vitality to the brain and nerve cells, to feed the

muscle cells, and to provide body energy. Oxygen is taken by the metabolic system and promoted into the blood to help improve youthful health. During a one-day "all liquid" controlled fasting program, live food juices help put life into the sluggish metabolism, promoting youthful vitality.

2. *Puts Youth Back into Digestion.* A rested and refreshed digestive system rewards you with a feeling of youthful functioning. Live food juices during a controlled fasting program help in the enzymatic function in the entire organism, to improve digestion of food. By giving the digestive organism a rest from working on heavy foods, you help refresh-rejuvenate this system so that it can perform better in assimilation of enzymes. A well-rested digestive system means that the digestive tract, the liver, the kidneys, the gall bladder, and the intestinal tract will all benefit from a brief "vacation" and be glad for the cleansing benefits of the live food juices. Live food juices then become absorbed from your digestive tract into your blood and lymph to create overall nourishment. Your bloodstream carries the absorbed nutrients from live food juices to the tissues and gathers up the end products of metabolism. All this is done better and faster when the digestive system is given a brief respite from churning solid foods in the digestive process and refreshed through a controlled fasting day with live raw juices.

3. *Gives Respiration a Breath of Refreshment.* An over-worked respiratory system chokes off the efficiency of the body's breathing. One day of liquid foods helps give the respiratory system a refreshing breather of rest. During controlled fasting, nutrients in raw juices enter into the bloodstream which carries oxygen to all body cells and carries away the waste products. A refreshed-relaxed respiratory system brings air from the external environment to the lungs to be circulated throughout your body. Your blood carries the carbon dioxide by-product back to the lungs to be exhaled. By devoting one day to liquid foods, you permit the respiratory system to perform its life-and-breath function with greater ease and relaxation. The billions of body cells and tissues enjoy refreshing "aeration" because of this pause that refreshes!

4. *Puts Youthful Color into Your Circulation.* The circulatory system has been called the "river of life," the "life blood," or the "life force." This is all too true when we see that the circulation influences the youth of the heart, the blood, and the blood vessels. The circulation is a system of perpetual motion, a two-way lifeline, coursing through your body in never-ceasing activity. A problem is that excessive over-eating often puts such a strain on the circulatory system that it breaks down under the pressure. During a one day all-liquid controlled fasting program, the bloodstream is able to carry the oxygen and nutrients throughout the body, to feed all glands to promote "happy hormones." A relaxed circulatory system that works at happy normalcy is beneficial for the heart. The alternate contracting and relaxation of the rings of the heart muscle causes the action that propels blood throughout the entire system. A youthful circulation enables the heart to function properly, maintain healthful blood tone, and a youthful color in your skin. A one-day liquid food fast gives rest to the circulation; this includes physical, mental, sensory, and physiological rest. Be good to your circulation and heart. They're made to last a lifetime!

5. *Improves the Vital Process of Elimination.* Liquid juices during a raw juice fast work with youth-restorative benefits upon the organs of elimination. In addition to the bowels, the other organs include the skin, lungs, and kidneys. All excrete water which is essential. Self-cleansing is possible when the elimination system is kept free-flowing and cleansed. Live food juices nourish the organisms so that the lungs can successfully excrete carbon dioxide, and the kidneys and intestinal organs can eliminate salts, nitrogenous substances, and food residues. Controlled fasting helps the entire "family" of elimination since each must work with the other. Constipation responds to all-liquid fasting since this distress is caused by the retention of waste residues beyond the normal period of a movement. A liquefying process helps improve digestion, absorption, and cellular metabolism. Raw juices are prime sources of vitamins, minerals, enzymes, and amino acids, that act upon sluggish elimination and promote a feeling of revival. Controlled live food juice fasting helps ease

problems of internal stagnation and promotes a young eliminative system.

How to Schedule a Raw Juice Fast Day in Your Look-and-Feel-Young Program. To benefit from "internal scrubbing," schedule one day per month to have a raw juice fast. You will find, as have so many countless others, that it helps promote a feeling of youth, an internal rejuvenation that gives you the look of a second youth. Just as your body requires eight hours of sleep nightly, so your internal systems require at least twenty-four hours of restful relaxation, once a month.

HOW JANE E. PLANS HER ONE DAY "ALL LIQUID" YOUTH RESTORATION PROGRAM

A bookkeeper, Jane E. manages to schedule one day per month for her controlled raw juice rejuvenation program. Jane E. usually picks the first Sunday of every month. Here is her program:

Morning: A special Flaxseed Cereal. Jane prepares it as follows: In two cups of boiling water, she stirs in slowly about one cup coarsely ground fresh flaxseed (available at most health stores) and one teaspoon kelp. She removes from fire. Covered, it steeps for five minutes. She now adds one cup chopped dates or raisins and one-half cup chopped nuts. Covered, it remains for five minutes to let all ingredients blend. Then she eats this with some honey and nut milk.

Luncheon: Two glasses of freshly squeezed root vegetable juices. Combinations of beets, radishes, and carrots are rich in minerals.

Dinner: Two glasses of freshly squeezed seasonal fruit juices, sprinkled with wheat germ flakes and some honey to add good taste.

Nightcap: Slightly heated apple juice to which one-half teaspoon cinnamon has been added. Has a relaxing effect on the body organs.

Benefits: The flaxseed cereal is brimming with seed oils

that promote a lubrication of the vital body processes. The added fruits offer vital energizing substances that are taken up by the bloodstream. The vegetable juices for lunch are dynamic sources of minerals needed to build strong bones and nourish the bloodstream. The fruit juices for dinner offer essential vitamins, minerals, and enzymes that promote a self-scrubbing action. The Nightcap is rich in soothing minerals that help promote a natural and healthful sleep.

Jane E. finds that this special one-day "All Liquid" Youth Restoration Program puts color into her cheeks, better flexibility into her limbs, a feeling of gentle comfort to her "insides" as well as giving more energy. She is able to go to work the next day with a spring in her walk and a smile on her face. She hopes to be able to devote two days per month to this inner-rejuvenation program.

HOW TO BEGIN A CONTROLLED FASTING PROGRAM

The day before, prepare yourself for the event. Get a good night's sleep. In the morning, avoid excess work. The key word here is *relaxation.* Give your metabolism a chance to perform its rejuvenation work without the need to provide super-power to extra-heavy physical activities. Let all activities be diverted to your *internal* requirements. Go about your daily tasks with a calm attitude. Avoid any circumstances that may increase respiration or tension. If you are in the midst of stressful situations, postpone your fasting for another day when you can benefit from external tranquility. During this one day, relax, read, listen to soothing music, chat with a friendly neighbor, or do simple and easy tasks. In so doing, you relax your body and permit your internal systems to work with relaxed effort.

HOW TO END A CONTROLLED FASTING PROGRAM

The very next day, eat a modest breakfast. The same applies to lunch and to dinner, as well. It is unwise and contradictory to go off on an eating binge and overload a system that is relaxed and soothed. One woman finds that on the day after her fast, she responds better by eliminating a solid food lunch and taking only vegetable juices. She makes the adjustment much easier with that simple "lunch juice" plan. Of course, when you return to solid foods, be sure to emphasize natural and wholesome foods. Eliminate unnatural, synthetic, bleached, processed, and commercial foods that are chemically saturated and contrary to good health. Always emphasize Nature and you will be on the road to the Look and Feel Young goal.

INDIGESTION IS RELIEVED BY ONE-DAY CONTROLLED FASTING. Lewis E., an overly tense accountant, suffered from recurring indigestion. He was the habitual taker of alkaline fizz powders, over-the-counter drugs, patent medicines, bismuth salts, and laxatives. He found that his indigestion worsened under this chemical onslaught. He heard that devoting one day to liquid foods could help his organism become refreshed-rejuvenated. He had tried everything else, so he tried this program.

Breakfast: A cup of hot water to which was added two tablespoons of honey and four tablespoons of brewer's yeast flakes.

Luncheon: A mixed vegetable cocktail with lecithin powder. He also added one tablespoon of desiccated liver powder.

Dinner: Beet-lettuce juice; carrot-cucumber juice.

Nightcap: Cup clear broth.

BENEFITS: The above one day program helped Lewis E. because the freshly squeezed liquids helped nourish the billions of body cells. Furthermore, they had a buffering action upon the digestive tract and helped ease his stomach-churning agony. The live juices required little digestive work (therefore giving his overworked digestive system a welcome opportunity to rest-rejuvenate) and were absorbed directly into the bloodstream. The phosphates of succulent fruit and vegetable juices acted to perform a tranquilizing benefit upon the stomach. It helped calm digestive muscle spasms; it also helped reduce the excess acid volume secreted by tension-provoked glands. Relief was possible through natural raw liquids.

Compromise with Nature Causes Recurring Stomach Spasms. Lewis E. was able to feel a rejuvenation of his digestion under this liquid food program but it was a short-lived victory. Lewis E. still lived a tension-filled work schedule; he ate heavily of spiced-fatty foods and disregarded many of the health programs that emphasized all-natural and wholesome foods. He soon endured recurring stomach spasms that became so painful that he required home confinement. Now he is under such sedation that his recovery seems hopeless and he will probably become enslaved to drugs and medications to ease his symptoms. Lewis E. tried to compromise with Nature and ended up as the loser.

THE YOUTH-RESTORATION POWERS OF JUICES DURING A CONTROLLED FASTING DAY. Without interference of solids, freshly squeezed juices exert these youth-restoration powers:

1. *Fruits.* Nutrients in fresh fruit juices act as cleansers and detoxifiers of the system. They seek to wash off and slough away debris in the system.

2. *Vegetables.* Nutrients in fresh vegetable juices act as rejuvenators, repairers, and rebuilders of the body. They are able to perform this cellular-tissue rebuilding when introduced into a fasting system that is free from conflict with solid food.

SOLAR ENERGY PROMOTES YOUTHFUL VITALITY. Since fruits and vegetables are grown in healthy soil (it is wise to purchase organically grown foods), they receive from the sunlight what is called a "natural cooking through solar energy." This is the secret of the succulent joy of fresh juices. They are rich in the natural elements offered by sunlight. These same raw juices are speedily assimilated during fasting, and the solar energizing elements are built into the basic systems of the body. This is one secret of the rejuvenation power and youth-restoration effect of a one day "all liquid" program.

It is estimated that within 17 minutes after drinking a glass of fresh raw juice, the nutrients become digested and assimilated, absorbed by the bloodstream and glands. They are then speedily used to perform regeneration-nourishment of the billions of body cells and tissues. The special benefit here is that during controlled fasting, this is done with little effort on the part of the digestive system. To those who have a weak stomach raw juices may well offer the key to healthful rejuvenation.

RAW JUICES OFFER HEALTH-PLUS. It is known that the living cell portion of foods (enzymes) is destroyed by heat; the starchy matter is made more soluble; fatty matter becomes a local irritant. Heat changes the fibrous matter from a natural state to a harsh one; the inorganic elements of fruits and vegetables are reduced from an organic combination to an inorganic condition. It is wise to take food as Nature created it. Live raw juices contain the valuable youth-building elements that are tampered with in processing and cooking. When introduced without the interference of other foods during a one day "all liquid" program, the nutrients work freely to help create youth-restoration.

RAW JUICES HELP CONSERVE YOUTHFUL ENERGY. Fresh fruit and vegetable juices are often more beneficial than eating the whole plant because so much energy is required for digestion of the entire plant. For those who have "weak digestion" or "tired stomach," it is good to help rebuild-rejuvenate through a day of fresh raw juices. This helps store up and conserve youthful energy and help invigorate the digestive organism.

Select Organic Food Plants. It is wise to select fruits and vegetables grown on organic soil. During digestion, the liver must detoxify, destroy or metabolize all foreign substances. When you eat plant foods that are saturated with chemicals, preservatives, artificial flavoring additives, and chemical colors, it means an extra burden upon the liver, not to mention a toxic residue that remains as a corrosive blemish upon the organ. Wherever possible, select organically grown plant foods.

START THE DAY OFF WITH ALMOND MILK. A one-day "all liquid" youth-restoration program made Edwin J. feel better, but not as much as he expected. He would drink a glass of room temperature milk for breakfast. This, he was told, was the cause of his partial restoration. Cow's milk, like meat, has too high a second-hand protein and requires a great deal of pancreatic enzymes for digestion. Some people find this distressful. Edwin J. was then told to drink a glass of almond milk.

How to Make Almond Milk. Almonds should be ground up on a home mill (available at health stores) or pounded to a powdery pulp. Then blend in with one glass of bottled spring water. Stir vigorously. Drink in the morning.

Edwin J. Enjoys Digestive Rejuvenation. With Almond Milk as a starter, Edwin felt better than ever before. The benefit of Almond Milk is in its protein supply. It feeds the vital organs and introduces a treasure of amino acids that are then released to nourish and rejuvenate the organism and promote a look and feel of youth. Edwin J. hopes to devote two days monthly to the special controlled fasting with live food juices, including Almond Milk.

How to Open the Way to Youth-Restoration with Live Food Juices. Relax your system and then initiate self-internal cleansing and nourishment through gentle juices. Of course, the body needs bulk. It is not necessary or desirable to live on juices alone. Raw salads are necessary to keep the digestive tract in good working order. Raw juices are likewise necessary to lubricate and rejuvenate the system. A balance with Nature will offer a treasured balance of health and a feeling of youth.

HIGHLIGHTS:

1. Rest-rejuvenate the internal systems through controlled fasting and a nourishment from live food juices.
2. Liquid fasting helps rejuvenate the five basic health systems.
3. Schedule a Raw Juice Fast Day as Jane E. did and enjoy a glad-to-be-young-and-alive feeling.

4. Begin and end a fasting program with the suggestions listed.

5. How indigestion was relieved with a one-day fasting program.

6. Solar energy in juices promotes youthful vitality at any age.

7. Raw juices help conserve youthful energy.

8. How Almond milk put a person on the road to youthfulness.

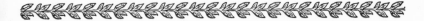

Chapter 20

How Herbal Teas Help Invigorate

Youthful Mind-Body Power

ALLEN E. thought he could increase his mental
output by drinking large amounts of coffee. As a production
supervisor in a large industrial plant, Allen E. needed a
combination of mental and physical power. For a while, the
endless cups of coffee made him energetic. Then he began to
develop nervous tremors. His vision blurred. His increasingly
rapid heartbeat worried him. When his fingers started trem-
bling and long columns of figures were swimming before his
eyes, he went to the company doctor for an examination. He
told of his "hard driving compulsion" that was propelled by
excessive coffee drinking. He was advised to eliminate coffee
and switch to herbal teas. It took a period of adjustment
before his respiratory-circulatory systems became stabilized.
Soon, Allen E. found that herbal teas provided a natural and
healthful mind-body energizer and he was able to work
overtime with none of his previous nervous symptoms. He

had "kicked" the coffee habit and learned that natural herb teas can boost the mind-body capacity to a healthful level.

WHY CAFFEINE-CONTAINING COFFEE SHOULD BE ELIMINATED IN THE QUEST FOR THE LOOK AND FEEL OF YOUTH. Caffeine-containing coffee is regarded as an unnaturally over-stimulating drink that whips up the action of the heart, nerves, and kidneys. This over-stimulation causes an emotional-physical drain that leads to premature depletion of youthful health. Caffeine adversely affects the higher centers of the brain. It may be responsible for problems of irritability, insomnia, and tachycardia (rapid heartbeat and corresponding fast pulsebeat, usually over 100 per minute).

Caffeine-Coffee is a Thief of Youth-Restoring Sleep. An authority has stated that definite impairment of sleep usually results from the consumption of an amount equivalent to six grains of caffeine, or about three cups of coffee. The blood pressure rises slightly and then falls, the pulse is usually accelerated and a diuresis (promoted excretion of urine) is evident. Insomnia is also traced to a vaso-dilation of the peripheral blood vessels, traced to caffeine in the coffee. Restless nights because of habitual coffee drinking is the penalty paid for this habit. Sleep is Nature's healing youth tonic and whatever interferes should be corrected. Caffeine in coffee is an unnatural substance and should be eliminated.

COMMERCIAL TEA CONTAINS CAFFEINE. It is known that tea leaves contain about twice as much caffeine as coffee beans. It is said that the drinking of excessive amounts of tea, especially if the leaves have been steeped for a long time, is a probable cause of dyspepsia (impaired digestion). Tea furthermore has a high purine content and its use is to be restricted in arthritic disorders such as gout. Commercial tea is subjected to harsh insecticides and sprays and their residue is often included in the beverage brewed at home.

WHY HERBAL TEAS ARE REJUVENATORS FOR THE MIND-BODY SYSTEM. Herbs are known for containing Nature-created ingredients that help promote a circulatory benefit to stimulate emotional and physical health. Most herbal teas have "nervine" qualities in that this ingredient lessens ir-ritability of the nerves and increases nerve energy. The tea is an infusion of the herb in hot water. The nutrients and Nature-created ingredients in the soil and plant are often found in the resulting tea. Caffeine-free, herbal teas introduce a gentle soothing benefit to the body and help promote youthful circulation that sends streams of fresh oxygen to the thinking centers of the brain. The reward is a fresh, clear-headed outlook and a youthful attitude toward the tasks of the day.

HERBAL TEAS OFFER THE PERFUME OF NATURE. Herbs offer a bouquet garden of scents that promote a perfume fragrance that is soothing and refreshing to inhale and taste-fully delicious to sip. Herb teas actually smell as good as they taste! Organically grown herbs have *natural* flavorful perfumes, in contrast to commercially grown teas which have chemicalized false scents added to delude you into believing they are natural. For the kiss-taste-scent of Nature, enjoy a garden of flavorful natural herbal teas.

HOW TO MAKE HERBAL TEAS. It is suggested that boiling water be prepared. Good spring or well water is best. Try to avoid chlorinated, fluoridated or otherwise chemically treated water from the tap. Use an earthenware pot, a porcelain or enamel pot, or an iron pot. Aluminum pots should be *avoided* since the heat has a corrosive action upon the porous con-struction and tends to release some of the aluminum by-products in the boiled water. Glass pots are the best.

Steep, Pour, Sip. Steep about one-half teaspoon of selected herbs for about five minutes. Then pour the herbal tea in a cup and sip slowly. Add honey to promote a natural sweet taste, if desired. For true bouquet and aromatic flavor, use fresh herb leaves. Some herbs are available in paper or cloth bags for convenience sake but they do not offer the complete natural perfume-flavor as the loose herb leaves. A warm cup of herbal tea is soothing to the digestive system and helps promote assimilation of nutrients that will refresh and invigorate the body and help create clear and youthful thinking.

HERBAL TEAS FOR MIND-BODY POWER

At an herbal pharmacy, select organically grown herbs for your teas. Here is a handy listing of reported herbs and how the natural aromatic teas have promoted remedial, restorative, and youth-rejuvenating benefits:

ADRUE. The ground root is used for making this tea. It has a bitterish, aromatic flavor of lavender. It creates a feeling of warmth throughout the system and promotes a natural tranquility upon the cerebro-nervous system.

AGRIMONY. Long used by the English and French, it has a nice sweet taste, promotes a gentle soothing action upon the circulatory system.

ANGELICA. It has a flavor resembling juniper berries. Its distinct flavor somewhat resembles that of old China tea. It is believed to ease nervous tremor and create clear-headed thinking ability.

BALM. Since time immemorial, balm has been used as a brew to make a tasty, flavorful tea to help increase emotional strength and give a youthful outlook. The English flavor it with a few flowers of lavender. Herbalists suggest that if some rosemary is added, it promotes the flavor.

BARBERRY. This is the ordinary barberry and the herbalists suggest that the berries be used to make a pleasant tea. It has a slight acid quality so it should be used in moderation.

BARLEY. Long known to be an excellent tea for the ailing. It promotes cellular rebuilding and this may be a reason for its use during convalescence.

CASSIA PODS. This tea has a high supply of Vitamin C and is said to have a "fruit laxative" action to help restore normal regularity without the need of harsh chemicalized cathartics.

CINNAMON. Has a delightful fragrance. It has the unique ability of being able to promote a feeling of refreshment.

COMFREY. Its taste is sweet, although it has little scent. Add lemon juice to promote its flavor. It is widely known to have nutrients and herbal ingredients that promote internal regeneration.

DANDELION. A tea is made from dried dandelion leaves, using one teaspoonful to one cup. It is said to be especially soothing for the internal organs such as the gall bladder and other vital parts.

DILL SEEDS. Herbalists say that dill seed tea is supposed to be an effective help in the case of hiccups. When dill seeds are combined with anise seeds, chamomile, and hop shoots, the tea acts as a natural sedative and promotes refreshing youthful sleep.

FENNEL SEED. The herbal tea made with fennel seed is said to nourish the cellular-tissue network and promote a healthful skin.

FENUGREEK. This tea has long been used by those who seek to improve the respiratory system. Proper aeration is said to promote clearer thinking.

FIG. Sun-dried figs can be soaked overnight in boiled water. Next morning, simmer the water and enjoy this fig tea which is both laxative and nutritive.

FLAXSEED. Take an ounce of whole flaxseed, a quarter teaspoon of honey and some lemon juice. Pour into a quart of boiling water. Let stand for several hours while it simmers. Strain off the tea. Its palatable taste is soothing and also helps promote a feeling of nerve relaxation.

GINGER. This is an old-time favorite used as a natural stimulant and invigorator and also for counteracting problems of chills caused by dampness or cold weather. In the West Indies, "medicine men" use it with a few cloves as a tea to help stimulate sluggish thinking.

GOLDENROD. Often referred to as Blue Mountain Tea, it has a gentle perfume. When brewed, it makes a delicious golden tea and has a warm anise-like flavor and fragrance. Pioneers would drink goldenrod tea when they wanted to improve their strength and their mental faculties.

HAWTHORN. This well-known plant whose berries ripen in September, has long been used in botanic medicine, especially for invigorating the heart. Its leaves are used in Europe, where it is said to help refresh-rejuvenate the heart system.

HOREHOUND. This herb tea offers a most agreeable flavor and makes a refreshing and healthful beverage. It is said to help relax the entire cerebro-nervous system and promote natural sleep.

HYSSOP. One herbalist said that hyssop tea with figs and honey would help chronic bronchitis and cough distress.

JUNIPER. This mountain healer was said to have a rejuvenating benefit upon folks of all ages.

LINDEN. Long a favorite in Europe, its bouquet flavor is rich with nutrients that promote natural relaxation.

LOVAGE. It is claimed that lovage tea has the benefit of an "internal bath" and promotes self-cleanliness and a feeling of internal rejuvenation.

MARJORAM. The tea is made from the herbs and leaves. It is regarded as a "youth tonic" among legendary herbalists and is known for promoting a healthful stimulation that gives the look and feel of youth.

MULBERRY. The fruit of the mulberry, when squeezed, and the juice extracted, makes a gentle tea. It is said to control thirst and also "cleanse" the bloodstream. Herbalists suggest taking mulberries, pouring hot water over them and then drinking the liquid as a tea.

PARSLEY. A highly nutritious tea, it contains antiseptic qualities and promotes a detoxification that helps promote a youthful feeling.

RASPBERRY LEAF. Used for centuries in Europe where legend has it that the tea promotes fertility in males and females. It has a delicious fruit flavor.

ROSEMARY. Was used many hundreds of years ago by people of the Mediterranean. It was said to clear up cases of headache. To prepare a legendary "mind building" tea, combine rosemary with lavender, add a bit of lemon juice and natural organic honey. Sip slowly.

SAGE. Sweeten with maple syrup or tea. It is claimed that the Orientals enjoyed "perpetual youth" with a sage tea.

SASSAFRAS. The bark of the root ground to a powder is usually used for this tea. Only a quarter teaspoonful is needed to make a cup. It is said to have mental-stimulant qualities.

SENNA. The flavor is somewhat sweet. When combined with other aromatic and stimulating herbs, it has a gentle internal-washing benefit. Herbalists report that senna tea is able to promote a feeling of youthful invigoration.

THYME. This tea gives off a good flavor when served with lemon. It is said to stimulate blood circulation and help promote warmth in the fingers and toes. Herbalists always prescribed thyme tea for the aged who benefited with a young-again feeling in their improved circulation.

WINTERGREEN. This rose-colored tea has its own natural sweet flavor and needs no honey. It offers a pleasant lingering after-taste. It is said to be a valuable folk healer for arthritis disorders and also promotes a youthful metabolism-digestion.

YARROW. Distinctly used as a medicinal brew by the folk herbal practitioners. Used as a beverage by Swiss mountaineers who claim it gives them such youthful strength of limbs and clear thinking, it may well be a fountain of youth! It has a bland scent and if combined with elder flowers, peppermint and honey, it offers a fragrant brew. Also said to help build resistance against influenza, colds, bronchial disorders, and winter ailments.

Enjoy Renewed Youthful Health with Herbal Teas. Select organic herbs from a reputable herbal pharmacy and enjoy renewed health with teas made from Nature's grasses. These natural beverages contribute to the pleasantries of living with their exotic aromas, fragrances, bouquets, tangs, essences, pungencies, and balsamics. This flood of youthful redolence is set free by the mere addition of boiled water. Many of these teas have been used throughout the ages, all over the world, for curative, therapeutic, remedial, restorative, and health-youth purposes. They are available today for your use to help promote the look and feel of youth with renewed health.

HIGHLIGHTS:

1. Commercial coffee and tea contain caffeine which is said to adversely affect the mind-body functions. This unnatural influence is detrimental to the look and feel of youth.

2. Herbal teas are reported to be rejuvenators of the mind-body system.

3. Select favored herbs from a reputable herbal pharmacist and drink your way to Nature's restored youth.

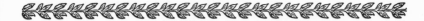

Chapter 21

Your Home Guide to Fruit

and Vegetable Juices

FRESH raw juices and liquid foods furnish the spark to ignite the flame of the look and feel of healthy youthfulness. When liquids are used as the foundation for rebuilding health, there should be a benefit of increased vigor, resistance to recurring symptoms, and gradual improvement of basic health and appearance. You have all of Nature's powers behind you when you take advantage of the garden of youth in Her fresh raw fruits and vegetables. The juices may well be likened unto the mythical Fountain of Youth. These springs of health burst forth from fruits and vegetables and bring about their soothing benefits and help promote hope for the look and feel of youth.

There is a wide variety of Nature's foods available to suit taste and individual requirements. In each of Nature's foods there are valuable nutrients that reportedly help cleanse-repair-recharge the body and mind with living health. Here is a listing of foods in Nature's garden of youth:

ALFALFA JUICE. Ancients hailed it as "green gold." It is a good source of minerals including phosphorus, calcium, chlorine, and magnesium. It is known to be a good alkalizer and has a high protein content. A good source of many essential amino acids which regenerate skin and body tissues.

APPLE JUICE. A prime source of such minerals as iron, silicon, and magnesium. Rich in potassium to help promote youthful metabolism. A good supply of maltic acid which is known to soothe internal inflammation.

ARTICHOKE JUICE. An amazing source of phosphorus and iron that becomes hydrolized to levulose during digestion to produce youthful vitality. It has bone-strengthening manganese, as well as valuable Vitamins A and C.

ASPARAGUS JUICE. Grows deep in the soil and the roots suck up valuable minerals. The sunshine then nourishes the tips as they emerge from the soil to promote its green juice. Has a soothing effect upon the system and promotes waste removal. Highly nutritious are asparagus with unbroken tips and meaty-thick stalks.

BEET JUICE. A good source of natural sodium and other minerals. Its calcium, potassium, iron content helps nourish the bloodstream. Known to youthfully stimulate the circulatory system's lymphatic flow. The leaves are iron-rich sources. Fresh beets are more flavorful.

BROCCOLI JUICE. A member of the cabbage family, this Nature food offers a variety of vitamins and minerals. Helps maintain a youthful bloodstream and a healthy circulation.

CABBAGE JUICE. Contains enormous amounts of Vitamin A as well as many minerals. Soothing to the digestive organs, especially the peptic tract. Many report treating and healing stomach ulcers with cabbage juice.

CARROT JUICE. Prime source of Vitamin A which is needed for visual health. Also rich in minerals which promote strong internal cleansing. Nutritionists inform us that carrot juice has an iron-calcium supply that is almost completely utilized by the weakest of systems to promote regeneration.

CELERY JUICE. Select very green celery for more nutritious value. Green leaves contain Vitamin A. The stems have the B-complex and C vitamins. Celery juice reportedly soothes stomach and heart. Its mineral content helps control nervous disorders. During juicing, nutrients are released from the crude fiber or cellulose. A glass of fresh celery juice is said to promote natural ventilation and maintain a cool temperature during hot spells.

CUCUMBER JUICE. A strong supply of vitamins, especially skin-building Vitamin C. Also has high mineral supply that helps relieve metabolic distress. Rich supply of magnesium to promote a feeling of coolness and relaxation.

ENDIVE JUICE. Helps promote regular elimination and is said to contain minerals that soothe and ease the digestive system and nourish the liver. It has a rather tangy taste so add to carrot or celery juice for a healthful youth cocktail.

KALE JUICE. A strong supply of Vitamin A and minerals. Used by the British during wartime rationing and found to have admirable nourishing qualities.

LEMON JUICE. A rich bioflavonoid source. Its high Vitamin C supply helps build skin and tissue capillaries. Also rich in minerals. A supply of hesperidin in lemon juice is Nature's gift because this substance helps the body utilize Vitamin C. During juicing, the hesperidin is released. It helps neutralize acid metabolism in the system and promote digestive youthfulness.

LETTUCE JUICE. A rich mineral supply (especially of magnesium), this juice helps youthify the powers of the nerves, brain, and muscular tissues. Magnesium in lettuce juice participates in regeneration of nerve and lung cells. The ancients would use lettuce juice to treat insomnia, fatigue, and weakness. Many regard lettuce juice as a natural alkalizer to control problems of acidity. Select the dark green leafy variety.

MUSTARD GREENS. The juice of this vegetable is rather

strong, but combined with lettuce juice, it offers a refreshing and tasty combination. Good for rebuilding the health of the smallest veins with its high vitamin-mineral supply.

OKRA JUICE. Slim down and satisfy your appetite with okra juice which is low-fat and low-carbohydrate. Has a high mineral content. Has been found to be healing for intestinal and colitis disorders.

ORANGE JUICE. A marvelous source of Vitamin C. Highly recommended by leading nutritionists as a source of energy because of its all-natural sugar supply. Its bioflavonoid content helps promote vascular strength and oxygenate the brain to ease fatigue or problems of aging.

PEACH JUICE. The peach skin is a rich supply of vitamins and minerals. Juicing releases these nutrients to help build skin and tissue health.

PEPPER JUICE. The greener the pepper, the richer the supply of vitamins and minerals. Pepper juice is a prime source of silicon which is needed to feed hair and skin.

PINEAPPLE JUICE. A prime source of bromelin, an ingredient said to duplicate pancreatic secretions and thereby regarded as Nature's own "hormone tonic." Has enzymes that work upon foods to facilitate digestion and promote absorption. Rich supply of energy-producing sugars as well as health-building minerals.

PLUM JUICE. Good sources of Vitamins A, B-complex and C as well as silicon (called the "youth vitamin") and many minerals that invigorate and rejuvenate the blood system.

RADISH JUICE. A miracle source of potassium and magnesium, as well as iron. These minerals perk up appetite, improve digestion, and promote an antiseptic benefit upon the intestinal system. The prime sulphur content helps tone the bloodstream. Somewhat strong, radish juice should be taken with other vegetable juices.

STRAWBERRY JUICE. Put strawberry colors in your cheeks with this high iron source. Contains essential minerals that soothe internal rumbles. Myth has it that the ancients turned the fruit of the rose inside out and created the strawberry. Put roses in your cheeks with this fruit juice of the gods!

TOMATO JUICE. Has a delicately tart flavor and a gold color of health. *Unique benefit:* exerts a natural alkaline effect to help neutralize excessive acid conditions such as those caused by consumption of too many concentrated starches. A glass of tomato juice puts the healthy glow of youth into your stomach and makes eating a joy instead of a threat.

THREE BENEFITS OF LIVE FOOD JUICES
FOR ADDED YOUTHFULNESS

1. *Solves Poor Chewing Problems.* People who have difficulty chewing will find live food juices an excellent way to drink their vitamins and minerals with little effort except swallowing. This promotes feeling and looking more youthful.

2. *Appeals to Fussy Eaters.* Many fussy eaters dislike some fruits and vegetables and won't eat them! But live food juices offer a delicious way to drink your vegetables—even those vegetables you ordinarily dislike, take on a zesty flavor when offered in the form of a bubbly cool juice.

3. *Nature's Endless Variety of Taste.* If you have certain tastes and like some vegetables but dislike others (the same applies to fruits), then juicing them at home offers you an endless variety of taste thrills. Some people who just can't stand carrots will enjoy carrot and lettuce juice in combination. Others who dislike apples will thrill to them when the juice is mixed with pineapple and pear juices. Disguise flavors and discover new exotic tastes with juice combinations. If you dislike eating salads—*drink them!*

Fresh live juices are brimming in Nature's succulent vitamins, minerals, enzymes and amino acids, waiting to help you to youthful health. All this is yours for the drinking!

YOUTHFUL HEALTH IS YOUR FIRST WEALTH. Centuries ago, the Grecian philosophers described health as a person's most precious gift. Today, we call health—the "first wealth." Good health is an active state of youthful physical and mental well-being. It is the ability to function fruitfully. Cultivate this ability with good, natural living programs and fresh raw life-food juices in the drinks described in this book. With good health customs, physical fitness, adequate sleep, a nutritional approach to long life, regular physical examinations, and with an alliance with Nature, you will be rewarded with the added look and feel of youth. It will be the greatest and the best wealth you need to possess.

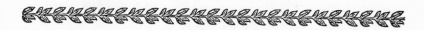

Index